FARRELL

THE STORY
OF
BLINDNESS

THE STORY

OF

BLINDNESS

Gabriel Farrell

HARVARD
University Press
Cambridge

© COPYRIGHT 1956

BY THE PRESIDENT AND FELLOWS OF HARVARD COLLEGE

SECOND PRINTING, 1969

Distributed in Great Britain by

OXFORD UNIVERSITY PRESS: LONDON

SBN 674–83940–4

Library of Congress Catalog Card Number 56–7212

PRINTED IN THE UNITED STATES OF AMERICA

Preface

THE main part of this volume constituted the Lowell Lectures, delivered in Jacob Sleeper Hall, Boston University, during November 1953. Since then, the lectures have been considerably revised and amplified to include material ruled out by the inexorable fifty-five-minute period allowed for each of eight lectures. Originally bearing the title "Social Aspects of Blindness," the final manuscript had so far transcended that limitation that the present title, "The Story of Blindness," is a more comprehensive description.

In trying to tell the story of blindness, my purpose has not been to extol those who carry on with spirit and success when sight is impaired, although for them we must have the highest respect, nor to bemoan the fate of those who seem unable to rise above their physical handicap, and for whom we cannot escape responsibility; but to tell those who still enjoy the full benefit of sight that they have a responsibility for that segment of society which is without sight. The burden rests the more heavily upon the sighted when it is realized that fully one-half, and perhaps three-quarters, of blindness could be prevented by appropriate medical and social services. And if a sense of social responsibility for those without sight is lacking, we may well strike at self-interest—for it may happen to you. The National Society for the Prevention of Blindness states that at least 750,000 Americans now living will be overtaken with blindness.

In preparing this book for publication, I have tried to select and present from the vast amount that has been written about blindness enough to show attitudes toward those without sight and to relate the efforts of many, both institutions and individuals, in all parts of the world, to alleviate the condition of the blind and to reduce its crippling consequences. If in citing institutions there may seem to be a tendency to refer too often to the school with which I was associated, insularity is not entirely the reason. For I found, as did Richard S. French when writing *From Homer to Helen Keller,* that

Perkins Institution and Massachusetts School for the Blind, by reason of the voluminous reports of its first superintendent and because of the great publicity given it, has by far the most complete and satisfactory records. Without intentional slight to the institutions in New York and Philadelphia, it may be best to follow the history of the New England Institution for the Education of the Blind, as it was originally called, with a view to seeing what was typical in its early growth and also to understand certain movements on behalf of the blind that had their beginnings in this more than in any other institution. In Boston, too, and later in Watertown, there has always been a very clear conception of educational ends, which, coupled with the long tenure of the superintendents and the unbroken continuity of effort toward those ends, makes the institution in large measure the norm for judgment of the work of other institutions.

And also if there may seem to be too many references to Samuel Gridley Howe, it is not a matter of partiality, but rather of authority. For it is beyond question that his fertile mind and humanitarian spirit made him stand far above all others. When Edward E. Allen, a successor of Dr. Howe and my immediate predecessor at Perkins, was asked to name the ten outstanding leaders in the field of the blind in America, he listed nine and then concluded:

Samuel Gridley Howe, pioneer and original first cause of many movements and inventions; maker of the Roman line type which took the first prize in the World's Fair of London in 1851; sane prophet of the future of the blind; promotor of the idea that their diffusion in society is their salvation; writer of our most philosophical reports on the education of the blind. Where Howe sat was ever the head of the table!

In making the acknowledgments customary in a preface, I wish first of all to express my deep gratitude to Ralph

Lowell, Trustee of the Lowell Institute, for inviting me to join the distinguished company of scholars who through one hundred fourteen years have been giving the public lectures made possible under the will of John Lowell, Jr. This invitation tied me down, as I told Mr. Lowell at the time, to put in writing the knowledge of the blind acquired through twenty years as Director of Perkins Institution. During these years, opportunity to learn ranged from daily contact with blind children to participation in national and international conferences dealing with the problems of blindness. I would also thank those who faithfully came to the several lectures and patiently heard them through. The lectures were also made available to larger audiences when broadcast over Station WGBH–FM. As a result of both mediums, I received many pleasant and informative comments, for which I am most grateful.

Following the broadcast of the lecture in which I intimated that a possible reason for Samuel Gridley Howe's determined decision to go to Greece to take part in the revolution of the Hellenes was due to the fact that he had been jilted by a Boston young lady, I received a telephone call from a woman who assured me that that was true. She remembers well, she said, her grandmother often telling of "that foolish Hap Howe who jilted the distinguished and wonderful Dr. Howe. With her trousseau complete and the wedding plans all made, she ran off with another man named Howe but not related to the great Dr. Howe." And to reveal the wide range, I must add that when one of my sons and his wife were listening to one of the broadcasts their three-year-old daughter playing nearby suddenly looked up and said, "That sounds like Button" (her name for her grandfather). Going closer to the radio, she listened for a moment, then walked away saying, "He doesn't make any sense! "

I want to express appreciation to Edward J. Waterhouse, Director, and to the Trustees of the Perkins Institution for the privilege of delving into the rich store of invaluable material deposited in the special blindiana library, the greatest collection of material on the blind in the world, and also to Edwin B. Dunphy, chief of ophthalmology, and to the managers of the Massachusetts Eye and Ear Infirmary for the opportunity to seek material in their medical library. In the latter library, Charles J. Snyder was most helpful, and at Perkins, Nelson Coon, the librarian, contributed greatly by digging out material long buried and not previously published. Dr. Franklin M. Foote and Miss C. Edith Kirby of the National Society for the Prevention of Blindness are deserving of thanks for reviewing the chapters on medical aspects of blindness, an area in which I lack competence to speak with authority.

Dr. Leona Zacharias, research worker for the Foundation for Vision, was most helpful in my effort to tell in simple terms the perplexing problems of retrolental fibroplasia, the new disease found in children prematurely born which has reversed the downward trend in childhood loss of sight. Charles C. Ritter of the American Foundation for the Blind and Dr. Clifford M. Witcher of the Massachusetts Institute of Technology were helpful in checking the technical aspects of the chapters on devices for the blind. And last but by no means least, my unbounded thanks to my wife and daughter, who patiently read the manuscript to see that the *i*'s were dotted and the *t*'s crossed and other changes introduced to make the text more readable. If mistakes or obscurities are found, the blame is mine, for I did not always accept suggestions for changes. My chief regret is that so many institutions have been omitted and innumerable deserving persons have not been mentioned. Here again the space limitations of a readable book have proved to be as inexorable as the time factor with the original lectures.

G.F.

Contents

THE STORY
OF
BLINDNESS

1 SHOOTING STARS
ON THE HORIZON

BLINDNESS is becoming a social problem sharply impinging on the conscience of the world. Aware that more than half of the persons now blind need not have lost their sight or could have had their visual disabilities corrected, society can no longer ease its concern by the old medium of the tin cup nor by the more modern method of pensions and relief. Even if a person is incurably blind, he still has social rights and economic possibilities that must be realized and fulfilled. This calls for the clarification of the many aspects of blindness and the determination of the measure of society's responsibility for that segment of the world's population which labors under the handicap of visual impairment.

The modern world is becoming increasingly conscious not only of the problems confronting its citizens of the dark but also of the potential contribution to society that can be made by the sightless. It must be remembered that human blindness is as old as life itself. And from the earliest times blindness has aroused compassion, based primarily on two almost conflicting emotions: fear and sympathy. Fear, not of the blind but that their own sight might be lost, engenders in people a sympathy that makes them want to help the blind and to make life as easy as possible for them. This urge to help takes many forms and covers a wide range.

In the Bible, concern for the sightless extends from the negative injunctions of the Old Testament, "Thou shalt not put a stumbling block before the blind," and "Cursed be he that maketh the blind to wander out of the path," to the more positive approach of the New Testament, which reports that blind Bartimaeus came to Jesus asking not for alms but for the restoration of his lost sight. While Bartimaeus expressed a universal hope for the restoration of sight, it must not be overlooked that when Jesus came his way he was sitting by the gate begging. In those days, that was normal for the sightless.

People may scoff at blind beggars, but it must not be forgotten that begging at that time was not entirely due to destitution, but was also the outlet for the compassion of seeing people who wanted to help the sightless. The gates in the city walls and the steps of the churches, considered choice locations for begging, were reserved for the blind by common consent. And in many of the socially backward countries this is true today. Almsgiving of this type symbolized the community's sense of responsibility for the blind. In its way, it was the Social Security of its time.

Of course, not all of the blind of early days shared in the choice locations sanctioned for begging or benefited by the compassion of the seeing for the sightless. The great majority had no occupation and no source of income. Many, estranged from their families and rejected by society, lived their lives in loneliness and in wandering, and through the Middle Ages became a scourge in Europe and Asia. From this group, however, there emerged some who made such a deep impression on society that their names are still remembered and their achievements cited in various fields of endeavor.

Outstanding were the blind bards or wandering minstrels who went from court to court, from country to country, singing "strains divine" as the blind Homer indicates in his poem (Odyssey VIII) featuring the blind singer, Demodocus, who seems to reflect his own feelings regarding blindness.

> Call, too, Demodocus, the bard divine,
> To share my banquet, whom the gods have blest
> With powers of song delectable, what theme
> Soe'er his animated fancy choose.

And now the herald thither led with care
The tuneful bard; him partially the muse
And dearly lov'd, yet gave him good and ill;
She quench'd his sight, but gave him strains divine.[1]

There were many blind bards in the Homeric tradition, some equally picturesque if not as great; and many better authenticated, even if not as well known. Such a bard was Ossian, the son of the Caledonian hero, King Fingal, who lived about A.D. 300. Reputed to have lost his sight in battle, he wandered about the countryside playing a harp and singing songs of battle and of man's freedom.

I often fought, and often won, in battles of the spear.
But blind and tearful, and forlorn I walk with little men!
O Fingal, with thy race of war, I now behold thee not.[2]

Some feel that the earliest blind bards were among the Chinese, but the first record is not found until the seventh century, when it is known that blind men with "gong and song" were wide disseminators of folklore. At about the same time, the Japanese blind were recorders of history, reciting on request chapter and verse of annals of the past. In France, itinerant singers accompanied themselves on violins; in Rumania, shepherds' pipes were used; and in the Ukraine, the bards sang in public houses at the crossroads of the steppes. In Spain, the blind usually gathered at church ceremonies and were famed for their religious songs, and in Armenia, Georgia, and Czechoslovakia, sightless minstrels were sought for weddings, where their talent for improvisation was greatly appreciated. In nearly all countries, Christian, Moslem, and Buddhist, the blind bards, often led by a dog with a bell at its neck to herald their arrival, found favor as they sang the praises of the countries' heroes and of the ruling kings.

The publication of books, and more travel, doomed this way of life for the blind bards, for people lost interest in their entertainment and their lore. The last of the blind minstrels in the ancient tradition was Torlogh O'Carolan. Born in 1670, this genial but sightless son of Erin traveled from estate to estate, strumming his harp and singing songs of folklore, and was welcomed wherever he went. Torlogh, before his death, composed in the Gaelic tongue over 200 songs of love and of war which became widely known. Tom Moore, the Irish poet, adapted and published ten of these poems. When asked about his skill in music, Torlogh O'Carolan used to say, "My eyes have been transplanted to my ears."

Through the centuries, occasional blind persons were able to pull themselves out of the sea of illiteracy and to rise to great heights in several fields of endeavor. Outstanding among the great intellects of all time is Didymus, who followed Origen as head of the Catechetical School at Alexandria. Born in A.D. 308, Didymus lost his sight when about four or five years of age. He stands out, not only for his great learning, but also because he achieved success by his own devices. He carved out of wood an alphabet of letters and from them learned to form words and to construct sentences. This skill opened the way to learning and enabled him to acquire the great scholarship that he attained.

The development of high intellect and scholarly attainment among those who could not see was not considered possible at that time. But the indomitable spirit of this youth in Alexandria made him determined to possess wisdom. Didymus was so insatiable in his quest for knowledge that he exhausted those whom he engaged to read to him. With such help, he delved into the literature of his time, became well versed in philosophy, pondered in the field of theology, and even ventured into the areas of geometry and astrology. Meditating deeply on all that was read to him, Didymus became the great teacher of that era and his fame attracted to him aspiring scholars from many lands.

Didymus was great not only for the wisdom he possessed but also for the impression that he made upon his time indirectly through the influence exercised by his pupils and admirers. Tyrannius Rufinus, Latin theologian, who lived as a monk on the Mount of Olives, said of Didymus, "He applied himself not to reading but to hearing, in order that he might transfer those things to others." Palladius, pupil of Didymus and a Greek scholar who became a bishop in Asia Minor, expressed the opinion that blindness was a great blessing to Didymus, since by shutting out all distractions he could concentrate on his studies. It was through St. Jerome, however, that Didymus exercised his widest influence, for this pupil became one of the great doctors of the early church, translator of the Vulgate and author of many ecclesiastical works. From Jerome come most of the facts that are known about Didymus, of whom he wrote with "a touch of awe," marveling that a blind man could inspire so many scholars of the Church.

Another blind person whose story rises from the mythical into the historic is St. Hervé, the patron saint of blind musicians. He was born in a little village in Brittany, the son of a bard and a pious mother who became a Christian. Tradition presents him as a sightless, barefooted man who, led by a white dog, wandered through the byways teaching children to love God, their neighbors, and their daily work. There is, however, historic proof that the blind Hervé did found a small monastery in Brittany. After his death in 565, it became the shrine of blind musicians, and even now on June 2, the Feast of St. Hervé, they bring their instruments there for a blessing by their patron saint.

In far-off, and at that time isolated, Japan, there lived a blind person whose influence set a pattern for the sightless which differed from that in any other country and saved his land from the scourge of beggary. Born in 843, Prince Hitoyasu, son of the Emperor Ninmyo, lost his sight in his twenty-eighth year. Well versed in the Japanese and Chinese literatures and with a deep interest in music, he was, as a young man, appointed the governor of two provinces. Upon the loss of his sight, which was attributed to grief over the death of his beautiful wife, Prince Hitoyasu turned his attention to the blind and gathered many into his court.

At parties held at his palace in Kyoto, then the capital of Japan, the Prince took delight in sharing in the music of his new friends and in reciting poetry. Provision for alms to be distributed among the needy sightless, which the Prince inaugurated, was continued after his death and extended to the blind all over the country by successive emperors. Two fields of work, music and massage, were reserved for the blind; this work gave them economic security and has continued to do so to the present time.

Turning from a Buddhist, consider one who achieved greatness within the Moslem fold. Abdu'l Ala al Ma'arri was born near Aleppo in the year 973. At the age of four he lost his sight from smallpox. Determined to become a scholar, he memorized the contents of the three libraries at Haleb, Antioch, and Tripoli. In 1008, he visited Baghdad where he was honored by the poets of the fabulous city. After hearing the free-thinking scholars of that center of learning, he become a skeptic and renounced all religion.

During the lifetime of Abdu'l Ala al Ma'arri, Persia, liberated from Arab rule, was on the verge of the revival that led to her era of glory, and in the field of Arabic poetry of the time, Will Durant states, Abdu'l Ala "marked the zenith." [3] Instead of writing about women and war, as did most of the bards of his time, this poet discussed such profound subjects as "Is life worth living?" and "Does God exist?" In most of his poems, his skepticism is revealed:

> O fool, awake! The rites ye sacred hold
> Are but a cheat contrived by men of old,
> Who lusted after wealth, and gained their lust,
> And died in bareness,—and their life is dust. [4]

Two men of greater faith whose achievements came after their vision was impaired, were Prospero Fagnani in Italy and John Milton in England. They lived at about the same time and lost their sight at the same age, forty-four, but their careers were quite different.

Prospero Fagnani, one of the outstanding canonists of the Roman Church, was born in Italy at an uncertain date around 1590, but there is record that he died in 1678. At the age of twenty-one, he had attained the degree of doctor of civil and canon law and at twenty-two became secretary of the Congregation of the Council, which position he held for fifteen years. His loss of sight did not deter him from continuing his canonical studies and from writing his distinguished *Commentary on the Decretals of Gregory IX.* The first edition, in six quarto volumes, was published in 1661. Containing interpretations of the texts of the different edicts of Pope Gregory, the work is renowned for the clearness with which the most complex and disputed questions of canon law are explained. Benedict XIV gave this work his highest praise, and it gained for its author the title of Doctor Caecus Oculatissimus—"the blind yet most far-sighted doctor."

Perhaps because of his blindness, Dr. Fagnani cited with particular care the laws of the Church pertaining to the blind. According to the canons of the time, the blind, orphans, widows, and the aged were classified as "miserable" persons, and for that word in the text there seems to be no other adequate translation. From persons in this category the Church expected nothing. They need not pay taxes nor make contributions to the Church. The Church, Fagnani pointed out, does not mean to imply that blindness indicates mental disability, for it holds that the "blind in mind" are more to be pitied than the "blind in eye." And, the canonist states, those without sight should be treated like seeing people and helped according to their need rather than on the basis of their blindness.

Any account of outstanding blind persons would be incomplete without including John Milton, born in 1608. He, however, cannot be classified as a bard of the old tradition but as a great poet. Milton, like Fagnani, did not rise from the mass of the illiterate blind, for he had already achieved distinction when he lost his sight. Milton was graduated from Cambridge University where, although a brilliant student, he was in residence for seven years. This long period of study is now attributed to difficulty with his eyes.

Milton is interesting to students of blindness because he was so articulate about his own loss of sight. In the hope of help from the Royal Oculist at the court of Louis XIV, he wrote in a letter to Philarus, a Greek friend then in Paris, a detailed description of the symptoms leading to his impaired vision. This is considered by modern ophthalmologists to be one of the most revealing accounts ever written, though they do not agree on the cause of his loss of sight. In poems written during his blindness are many allusions that reflect Milton's reactions to his loss of sight. In *Paradise Lost,* he wrote:

> Thus with the Year
> Seasons return, but not to me returns
> Day, or the sweet approach of Ev'n or Morn,
> Or sight of vernal bloom, or Summer's Rose,
> Or flocks, or heards, or human face divine;
> But cloud in stead, and ever-during dark
> Surrounds me, from the chearful wayes of men
> Cut off, and for the Book of knowledg fair
> Presented with a Universal blanc
> Of Natures works to mee expung'd and ras'd,
> And wisdome at one entrance quite shut out.
> So much the rather thou Celestial light
> Shine inward, and the mind through all her powers
> Irradiate, there plant eyes, all mist from thence
> Purge and disperse, that I may see and tell
> Of things invisible to mortal sight.[5]

In other fields of activity blind persons have achieved greatness. In the field of mathematics there was Nicholas Saunderson, born in Yorkshire, England, in 1682. When a year old, he lost his sight completely from smallpox. His father undertook his early education and later sent him to an academy for seeing boys where he displayed unusual ability in mathematics. Much of this was done by mental calculation. In order to handle more complex figuring, Saunderson developed a ciphering board upon which he could work out mathematical and geometrical problems with lightning speed. A modified form is still in use in schools for the blind.

Saunderson was strong and forceful in seeking an outlet for his genius. When he had completed his schooling, a friend persuaded him to go to Cambridge, where he undertook private tutoring. His ability in mathematics was soon recognized and many students sought his help. Saunderson was not admitted to the University but was permitted to use the library. Later, however, the authorities allowed him to conduct a class on the principles of Sir Isaac Newton, who was then at the height of his fame. It was said that there were only twelve men in England at that time who understood Newton's *Principia* and Saunderson was one.[6]

Newton was so impressed with Saunderson that, when the chair which he had formerly held at Cambridge became vacant, he pressed for Saunderson's appointment. There was considerable opposition to the appointment because the blind man "had not matriculated at the University" and held no academic degree. The latter deficiency, however, was overcome by Queen Anne (who had recently knighted Newton) when she bestowed on Saunderson the requisite degree.

At the age of thirty, this blind man became the Lucasian Professor of Mathematics at the University of Cambridge, a post he held with distinction for nearly thirty years. In 1719, he became a Fellow of the Royal Society and in 1728, when George II visited Cambridge, he sought out Saunderson and made him a Doctor of Laws. One of his most popular series of lectures was on optics, which many felt a strange subject for a blind man. This caused the elegant Lord Chesterfield to comment on "the miracle of a man who had lost the use of his own sight teaching others to use theirs." Saunderson died in 1739 at the age of fifty-seven.

Consider another blind man of this period, John Metcalf, born in the north of England in 1717. Blinded at six, he led an active and independent childhood. Six months after his sight had gone, he ventured into the streets and when he was nine years old, he could go anywhere without a guide. He became a strong swimmer and acquired skill as a violinist.

At nineteen, Metcalf ventured farther afield, walking two hundred miles to London, visiting Windsor Castle and Hampton Court on the way. This he did in six days. He got about so freely that few thought of him as blind. Asked to take a stranger to Harrowgate, he agreed to do so on condition that the man was not told that he was without sight. When they arrived safely at their destination and the stranger learned that his guide was blind, he exclaimed: "If I had known your condition, I would not have trusted myself to you for a hundred pounds."

Not only in finding his way on bad roads but also in making them better Metcalf proved his genius. As a business venture, he set up a stagecoach service between York and Knaresborough and, disturbed by the way the coaches bounced on the rough roads, he determined to improve them. This led him into the road-building business, where he achieved great success. When a turnpike was to be built between Harrowgate and Boroughbridge, Metcalf put in a bid for a section and was awarded the contract. He encountered difficulty with a peat marsh but overcame it by crisscrossing branches and putting on layers of crushed stone. He was the first to use crushed stone in road building. Faced with the necessity for a bridge, he had his men dig nearby for rock and had the luck to unearth an old Roman causeway which provided the needed stone. In his lifetime, Metcalf constructed 180 miles of roads on contracts totaling £65,000.

Metcalf's life was not all work. In boyhood he was active in hunting and fishing. He became a proficient horseman and often entered races in which he followed the course by having someone stand near each post ringing a bell. He used a horse effectively in another way, for it is reported that Metcalf rode up to the inn in Harrowgate and snatched away one Mary Benson an hour before she was to marry another man. After that, it is recorded, they lived together happily for forty years. This genial blind man made life happy for others by the use of his fiddle, which he played at all the country fairs and feasts. At the age of ninety-three, John Metcalf died, leaving four children, twenty grandchildren, and ninety great-grandchildren.

Another intellectual blind man, this time a scientist in the interesting field of apiculture, was François Huber, born in Switzerland in 1750. He soon began to lose his sight from cataracts and was totally blind before his sixteenth birthday. François attended lectures at the University of Geneva, but because of poor health he was advised to live in the country. Here he undertook the study of bees, which he considered the most fascinating of God's creatures. By listening to their hum and recording their activities, he made profound discoveries about their life patterns.

Huber's work with bees was scientific and competent. He was the first to discover the nuptial flight, the bee's use of antennae, the genesis of swarms, and the true meaning of periodic migrations. By the time of his death in 1831, François Huber was recognized as the highest authority on the life and habits of bees. Maurice Maeterlinck wrote that Huber was "the master and classic of contemporary apiarian science . . . not a single one of his principal statements has been disproved, or discovered in error; and in our actual experience they stand untouched, and indeed at its very foundation." [7]

All of these people, however, were, as Michael Anagnos, the second director of Perkins Institution, pointed out nearly three-quarters of a century ago, "shooting stars on the horizon of deep darkness, ignorance, and neglect. The great mass of this afflicted class," he continued, "were everywhere mere objects of charity which, however wisely it may be administered, wounds the spirit while it soothes the flesh." [8] There is evidence, nevertheless, that these "shooting stars" were focusing attention on the sightless and here and there people were becoming concerned about their plight. The first book describing the condition and miseries of the blind was published in Italy in 1646, in the form of a letter to Vincent Armanni from "S. D. C.," who has never been identified. This was translated into French and apparently made a greater impression in France than in the country of its origin. In 1670, a book on the instruction of the blind was written by another Italian, a Jesuit named Lana Terzia.

In England also there arose a new interest in those who could not see. This, however, was not humanitarian, based on concern for the misery of the blind, but was pure speculation on a philosophical basis on such matters as whether or not a person who had never seen could, if sight were restored, recognize through seeing what he had learned to know through feeling. This discussion was touched off by the famous philosopher, John Locke, in his *Essay Concerning Human Understanding,* published in 1690.

Locke posed the question previously raised by the Irish member of Parliament and writer, William Molyneux, who claimed that a blind person on regaining sight would not recognize, through seeing, objects he had learned to know through touch. In this opinion, Molyneux was supported by Locke. Bishop Berkeley gave further stimulation to the discussion when, in his *Essay Toward a New Theory of Vision,* published in 1709, he maintained that, according to his philosophy, what one saw with his eyes was not sensations but inferences, not the immediate revelations of sight but the results of association and intellectual construction based on imagination and experience.

The belief that a blind person on recovering sight would not recognize objects with which he was familiar through touch gained scientific support when a thirteen-year-old boy operated on for cataracts by William Cheselden, an English surgeon, had his vision restored. With his new sight, the boy found it difficult to form any visual judgment regarding the shape of familiar objects. He was disappointed when he learned that the things and persons he loved best were not always the fairest to look upon. He had a hard time distinguishing between his dog and his cat. Being ashamed to ask the oft-repeated question which was which, he was observed one day passing his hand carefully over the cat and then looking at it steadfastly and saying, "So, puss, I shall know you another time." He had more confidence in the judgment of his hands than of his eyes.

People in England were not interested in the psychological aspect of Dr. Cheselden's report. It remained for the philosophers of France to exploit the case and to determine to carry the experiment further. Voltaire had already expounded Bishop Berkeley's new theory of vision, as he had previously promoted the principles of Sir Isaac Newton. Etienne Bonnot de Condillac, a younger man, in his *Essay on the Origin of Human Knowledge,* published in 1746, referred to the operation of Cheselden and discussed the effects of blindness on the power of perception. It was, however, the great encyclopedist, Denis Diderot, who brought the matter to an explosive head by his famous *Letter on the Blind for the Use of Those Who See,* published in Paris in 1749.

When Diderot heard of Cheselden's operation on the boy

in England, he resolved to observe a cataract operation and to make a similar study. This idea was not carried out, for he later decided to seek an average blind man and to learn his reactions to his loss of sight. In the little town of Puiseaux, Diderot found a blind man named Lenotre, the son of a professor in the University of Paris. After taking many courses in the University in chemistry and botany and running through his fortune, Lenotre had retired to the little town and established a distillery.

Lenotre coöperated with Diderot in his interview and gave carefully considered answers to his questions. He also raised some interesting questions for Diderot to answer, particularly about the use of microscopes and telescopes. When Diderot asked if he ever wished for his sight, Lenotre replied, "If it were not for curiosity, I would just as soon have long arms: it seems to me my hands would tell me more of what goes on in the moon than your eyes or your telescopes; and besides, eyes cease to see sooner than hands to touch. I would be as well off if I perfected the organ I possess, as if I obtained the organ which I am deprived of." [9]

Diderot's interest in the intellectual ability of the blind was later enhanced by his acquaintance with a young woman who had become a sensation in Paris. This was Mélanie de Salignac. Born in 1741 of a good family, Mélanie lost her sight at the age of two, when her mother "put pigeon's blood on her eyes to preserve them in the smallpox." This, however, was not successful, for the writer continues, "So far from achieving the end, it ate into them; nature, however, may be said to have compensated for that unhappy mistake, by beauty of person, sweetness of temper, vivacity of genius, quickness of conception, and many talents which certainly must soften her misfortune." [10]

When Diderot met Mélanie de Salignac in 1760, he was greatly impressed by her accomplishments, and in an addition to his famous letter, made some thirty years after the original, he tells how she had been taught to read by means of cut-out letters, and to write by pricking a piece of paper stretched on a frame. What she wrote in this way she read by passing her fingers over the reverse side of the paper. Diderot was also impressed by Mélanie's ability in astronomy, algebra, and geometry. He tells how her mother, after reading the Abbé de la Caille's textbook on geometry, would ask if she understood it. "Quite easily," she would reply. She declared, wrote Diderot, that "geometry was the science of the blind, because it was of such universal application and no external aid was necessary to become proficient in it. The geometrician," she added, "spends nearly all his life with his eyes shut."

I have seen the maps with which she studied geography. The parallels and meridians were made of wire; the boundaries of kingdoms and provinces of embroidery in linen, silk, or wool of various thickness; the rivers and streams and mountains of pins' heads of various sizes; and cities and towns of drops of wax of various sizes.

One day I said to her, "Mademoiselle, imagine a cube."

"I see it."

"Place a point in the center of the cube."

"I have done so."

"From the point draw straight lines to the angles; into what have you divided the cube?"

"Into six pyramids," she replied without hesitation, "each having as its base one side of the cube and a height equal to half its height."

"True, but tell me where you see this?"

"In my head, as you do." . . .

People will find it difficult to accept the following fact, though I and all her family, as well as twenty persons still alive, can vouch for it. Given a piece of poetry of twelve to fifteen lines, if she was told the first letter and the number of letters in each word, she could reconstruct the poem, however odd and far-fetched. I tried her with a poem of Colle's. She sometimes lighted on a better word than the original.[11]

In his *Letter on the Blind,* and in the addition published in his more mature years, Diderot made some profound observations. He advanced the opinion that the senses of the blind are not especially sharpened by the loss of sight, but that the loss of sight compels the increased use of the remaining senses; that education ought to be built on what the blind man has rather than on what he has lost; and above all else that he should keep active all possible contacts with the objective world. Even the deaf-blind, Diderot maintained, could be taught through touch by patient and insistent connection of tangible signs and objects.

The great value of Diderot's *Letter* was that, coming from such an erudite pen, it commanded the respect of the savants of the time, who through it came to know something of the sightless and their educational potentialities. The *Letter* also crystallized the speculations about the blind that were being discussed so commonly in the salons of the day. It focused attention not only on the blind who had achieved fame but also on the beggars still found at the doors of churches, the wandering bards common throughout Europe, and the misery of those who lived in darkness. The natural compassion of the seeing for the sightless was deeply stirred by these discussions.

2 BEGINNING WITH CHILDREN

"TRUE," wrote Michael Anagnos, "Diderot was the first writer who called special attention to the condition and wants of this afflicted class, and made them popularly known; but neither he, nor . . . any of the encyclopedists, went beyond the boundaries of abstract psychological speculation. They proposed no measures of practical utility or relief, nor did they devise any plans for the instruction and training of sightless people." [1] It took a younger man, one who had visited Diderot in prison and learned from him of the blind, to change speculation into a determination for action.

Jean Jacques Rousseau, soon to become the champion of humanity, whose "words, descending like a flame of fire, moved the souls of his contemporaries," gave expression to the hopes that had been aroused when he asked: "What can we do to alleviate the lot of this class of sufferers, and how shall we apply to their education the results of metaphysics?" [2] The humanitarian call of Rousseau led to action. Those whose interest in the blind had been aroused were learned men, so they turned naturally to education as the medium of alleviation. Schooling, they felt, based on senses other than sight, could surely be provided through the practical application of metaphysics. And so it happened that the earliest constructive work among the blind began with children.

The impulse to apply this principle came about in a most dramatic way. One of Rousseau's younger contemporaries, and one who had undoubtedly shared in the current philosophical speculations about the blind, their plight, and their possibilities, was sauntering down a street in Paris in September 1771. As he came to the Place Louis-le-Grand, now the Place Vendôme, his attention was attracted by loud hooting and laughter emerging from the Café Saint Ovide. Here a scene greeted his eyes which so revolted him that he resolved to devote his life to improving the condition of the sightless through the medium of practical education.

Mounted on a high platform in this café were ten blind men scraping crude bows on rough stringed instruments. Huge pasteboard spectacles devoid of lenses emphasized the emptiness of the sightless eyes. Lighted candles set to illumine the sheets of music only revealed their uselessness, for the notation was turned toward the audience. Grotesque robes and dunce caps with ass's ears added insult to the ridicule to which the men were subjected. For some two months, these poor beggars attracted business to the café by the discord they thumped out on the fake instruments as they moaned a monotonous chant. And in this burlesque at the expense of handicapped human beings, the Parisians of the time found amusement.

Not Valentin Haüy. Later, when reviewing this scene, he wrote:

Why was it that a scene so dishonorable to humanity did not perish the instant of its conception? Why was it that poetry and picture should lend their divine ministration to the publication of this atrocity? Ah! it was without doubt, that the scene reproduced before my eyes, and conveying to my heart profound sorrow, might inspire and arouse my soul. "Yes," I said to myself, seized by an exalted enthusiasm, "I will substitute the truth for this mockery, I will make the blind read. I will put in their hands volumes printed by themselves. They will trace the true characters and will read their own writing, and they will be enabled to give harmonious concerts. Yes, atrocious maligner, whoever thou art, the ears of the ass with which thou would'st degrade the head of misfortune, shall be attached to thine own." [3]

Valentin Haüy was born November 13, 1745, in St. Just les Marais, in Picardy, not far from Paris. His parents were

of the people, the father a weaver who supplemented his earnings at the loom by ringing the Angelus bell at the nearby
Premonstrant Abbey. Often Valentin and his older brother,
René, walked across the fields to toll the bell for their father.
In this way, they came to know the monks and under their
tutelage acquired a good education. René was brilliant and
was sent to Paris to the Jardin des Plantes to study botany
and mineralogy. Valentin soon followed and because of his
good training in languages secured work as a translator of
correspondence at the Ministry of Foreign Affairs, and in his
free time did some private tutoring.

René suddenly rose to fame because of his discovery, when
he accidentally dropped a bar of crystal, that each piece retained a constant form. This led to a new science, and his
lecture before the Academy of Sciences on crystallography
was widely acclaimed by the learned men of his time. This
gave René association with the great minds gathered in Paris,
then the intellectual center of the world, and in this the
younger brother shared. Through this association, Valentin
undoubtedly became acquainted with the discussions pertaining to the blind then current and learned of the writings of
Voltaire, Diderot, and Rousseau, who did so much to mold
the thought of that period and to brew the ferment which resulted in the French Revolution.

Haüy had also become interested in what was being done
for the deaf at that time. The pioneer work of the Abbé de
l'Epée with deaf-mutes was being widely discussed in Paris,
and the achievement of the Abbé Sicard, his successor, in
teaching one boy, Jean Massieu, communication through the
sign language commanded wide respect and strong support.
Haüy was impressed by this as he brooded upon the resolve
made at the time of the incident at the Café Saint Ovide.
More than a decade was to pass, however, before any active
steps were taken to "substitute the truth for this mockery."

Another incident strengthened Haüy's resolve and perhaps
gave a key to its solution. This was "a display of simple honesty on the part of a blind beggar. Given a coin larger than
he was accustomed to receive, the beggar called the donor

back and asked if he had not made a mistake. Haüy was impressed not only by the honesty of the man, but by his acuteness of touch. He began to consider the possibilities of a sense that could so readily distinguish the differences between two small coins." [4]

It took a woman, however, to get Haüy really started. The rage of Paris at that time was the fascinating Maria Theresa von Paradis, the blind pianist from Vienna. Born in 1759, she soon exhibited unusual ability, particularly in music. Her father, a councilor in the court of Empress Maria Theresa, was able to provide the best of tutors as well as to bring his child to the attention of the Empress. When the Empress heard Maria sing in the court church of Vienna, she arranged for lessons by a distinguished teacher and gave her parents an annuity of 200 florins to further her education. While concentrating on music, Maria studied languages, history, and geography, and acquired supreme grace and poise, so that she became a living example of what a blind person with education could do and be.

There is some difference of opinion as to the cause of Maria's blindness, and even its extent. When she was four, she awakened one morning with convulsive twitchings of her eyes so violent that "only the whites could be seen; at the same time, they protruded far out of the sockets." She was placed under the care of an Austrian oculist who for years tried to overcome the twitching, but it took the creator of mesmerism to have any effect on her blindness. Dr. Franz Anton Mesmer,[5] then at the height of his fame with his cult of animal magnetism, maintained that Maria's visual difficulty was due to shock and therefore was psychic. Putting her in a private nursing home, he began to treat Maria by waving his magnetized wand over her before a mirror. Soon all were convinced that her sight had been restored.

This caused considerable furore in the medical profession and a commission was appointed to investigate the claims. The members described Maria's cure as "a delusion, based merely on imagination" and asserted that "if she could see now, she had not been truly blind." The parents were frightened, partly because of the uproar and partly because it was reported that if Maria could see, the Empress would withdraw her pension; they also feared that her popularity as a pianist would decrease if she were not blind.

The parents asked Mesmer to give up his treatments. At first he was reluctant to do so, and when they resolved to take their daughter home, she refused to go, saying that she would continue to live in Mesmer's house and would never leave. Through a committee, appointed to sustain morality, Mesmer was forced to quit and Maria went home seemingly blind. To escape the excitement, her mother took her on a tour of Europe. The tour proved to be a triumphal progress. From one capital to another, Maria made her way, singing and playing in all of the courts of Europe.

In 1784, she reached Paris, where Queen Marie Antoinette became her sponsor. For some time the blind girl lived in the luxury of Versailles and gave concerts both there and in Paris. These were thronged by the great, who marveled not only at her musical achievement but also at her social charm as a blind person. The following winter Maria was in London, where at her concert in Covent Garden the Prince of Wales, later George IV, exclaimed: "Amazing! A blind girl! We must invite her to the palace." And the next night the blind girl from Vienna sang for the Royal Prince while he accompanied her on the cello.

Among those who attended Maria's concerts in Paris was Valentin Haüy. So impressed was he that he sought an audience and told her of his vow to educate the blind. Maria proved both helpful and encouraging. She told Haüy that she had learned to write by pricking out with a pin the letters of the alphabet on paper placed on a cushion and to read by reversing the paper and deciphering the pricked letters with her fingertips. She described a press that had been made for her which enabled her to print German characters in relief. But perhaps more important, she told Haüy of her correspondence with a young German named Georg Weissembourg, who, although blinded at five, had learned to read and write and had acquired considerable education. This youth had been fortunate in his teacher, Christian Niesen, who was clever in developing devices as well as in using those employed by Saunderson.

In a letter dated July 27, 1779, Weissembourg told Maria of his studies and of the maps and devices that he used. He said that he himself had taught an untrained blind boy the five branches of arithmetic in three months, adding,

Studies seem to clarify themselves and stick better when I expound them to another person; but what I am telling you here is merely to show you what we blind are capable of doing . . . If you care to enter a correspondence with me (a correspondence between blind persons is really a new phenomenon!) I shall gladly answer minutely in every particular and with all my ability . . . One must overcome all difficulties with patience and graciousness, though many hold them to be insuperable . . . and increase the little group of educated blind persons of whom you are one of the greatest.[6]

Here was the inspiration Haüy needed to fulfill the resolve that he had made fourteen years before when he was so deeply moved by the burlesque spectacle in the Café Saint Ovide.

Recalling the successful beginning that the Abbé Sicard had made through teaching Jean Massieu, Haüy began to look about for a youth of similar promise. On the porch of the Church of St. Germain, he found François Lesueur, then seventeen, illiterate, and without sight since he was six weeks old. At first, François was reluctant to give up his profitable spot for begging, since his large family needed all the money he could bring home. After persuasion from Haüy, Lesueur agreed to study afternoons if he were permitted to beg in the mornings and were paid for his afternoon losses. Soon the businesslike beggar became so absorbed in the experiment that he gave it his full time and attention, and undoubtedly Haüy made it worth while because of the success that they were achieving.

Having secured a promising pupil, Haüy then realized the need for educational media. He drew heavily upon the information given him by Maria von Paradis, investigated the maps and other appliances developed in the education of

Weissembourg, and made an improved model of Saunderson's mathematical slate. Haüy's greatest need was to find a medium of reading and writing without sight and this he attained in a way almost as dramatic as the incident at the Café Saint Ovide that had brought about his resolve to help the blind. It gave him further impetus to go on, for it provided the medium so greatly needed.

One day in 1786, François Lesueur, while handling some papers on Haüy's desk, accidentally ran his hand over a printed sheet. He passed his fingers over it again and then called the master. To him he pointed out the letter *o* which his fingers detected on what Haüy saw to be the reverse side of a funeral notice fresh from the press. This was the clue that Haüy needed. Away went the pricked letters of Maria von Paradis, the wooden blocks and metal slugs of Weissembourg. If François could distinguish letters so slightly raised in ordinary printing, what could any blind person do with enlarged type firmly and specially embossed. Soon Haüy was embossing sheets of paper with an italic script type commonly in use at that time. A way for the blind to read had been found!

With a medium of writing developed, his devices ready, and his methods formulated, Haüy began to make progress with François Lesueur. In six months, the blind youth could read and write embossed type. Confident in his progress, Haüy felt ready to ask for public approval and support. Through his brother René, now an accepted scientist in the scholarly circles of Paris, Valentin was given an opportunity to display his accomplishments and to demonstrate the progress of his pupil before members of the Royal Academy of Sciences. The learned men were deeply impressed and, after appointing a committee to make a further study of the venture, encouraged the younger Haüy to reach out and help other blind children.

To do this, Haüy had to secure the approval of the comptroller general, the keeper of the seals, and other government officials. Before them, he gave demonstrations that brought their approval. The additional pupils needed were fortunately found in a group of fourteen blind boys and girls under care as pensioners of the Philanthropic Society, which had recently been formed by some of the most distinguished men in Paris. The members were glad to have their wards become pupils of Haüy; in fact, the Society became the chief supporter of the growing school until the Revolution made away with the nobles who were its chief members.

The group of fourteen, with Haüy as head teacher and Lesueur as his assistant, were housed first in a dwelling on the Rue Coquilliere and later in the Rue Nôtre-Dame des Victoires. While still under the direction of Valentin Haüy, the school increased to fifty pupils and became known as L'Institution Nationale des Jeunes Aveugles (The National Institution for Young Blind People). Founded in 1784, it is recognized as the first school in the world for blind children.

To secure recognition and support for his school, Haüy set up the precedent, which still prevails in many places, of taking his pupils out to give demonstrations and concerts. Today this practice is defended on the grounds that it educates the seeing concerning the economic and intellectual possibilities of the well-trained blind. In Paris at that time, collections for the support of the school were taken after the demonstrations and this also has been known to happen in the United States. Haüy's pupils were asked to perform before many societies and the Royal Academy sponsored a concert for their benefit. During the Christmas festivities in 1786, the blind pupils and their master were invited to the court at Versailles, where they demonstrated their skills.

Queen Marie Antoinette, showing the same interest that made her mother, Empress Maria Theresa, the patroness of Maria von Paradis in Vienna, observed sympathetically these groups of blind children reading and writing, solving arithmetic problems, and working on their handicrafts. All were deeply moved when the pupils saluted the King and Queen with the "Ode to Heaven," sung for the first time at the concert sponsored by the Academy of Music. Three years later, unfortunately, Marie Antoinette went to the guillotine, and the King never awarded Haüy the Order of St. Michael promised at Versailles.

The Revolution, breaking into full terror, almost wiped out all that Haüy had done for the blind. But he was able to adjust himself and his school to the changing times. Many of his students became revolutionists, and he readily transferred his singers from chanting the offices of the Church to singing the songs of the Revolution. With his noble supporters gone, Haüy appealed to the Constituent Assembly, which in 1791 created under government auspices the Institution of Those Born Blind and moved Haüy and his pupils into the Convent for the Celestines, which they shared with a school for deaf-mutes. This was not a happy combination and it set an unfortunate precedent for dual schools in later years. In three years, however, the blind were moved to a house in the Rue des Lombards, their fourth home in ten years. Here the school reached a low ebb, for it became primarily a workshop and, in fact, its name was changed on July 28, 1795, to the National Institution of Blind Workers. Haüy struggled to keep the educational program alive and his printing press active, but lack of financial support and the shifting political forces made it almost impossible.

In October 1800, Napoleon moved all of the blind children to the Quinze-Vingts, an asylum reputed to have been founded by Louis IX for men blinded in the Crusades. Here they were classified as "blind of the second class." Those of the "first class" were the adult occupants of this asylum, numbering 300. Haüy was placed in charge of the 120 children. It was decreed that only totally blind children were to be admitted, at the age of seven, and that the educational program was to last for eight years, an age schedule still followed in many European schools. Napoleon, displeased with Haüy chiefly because of his political activities, dismissed him in 1802.

Haüy could not easily forget the blind to whom he had dedicated his life. Still resolved to help the sightless, he opened a small private school, which he carried on for only three years. During that time, however, he opened the way of education to two blind youths whose names became known throughout Europe. One, Alexander Rodenbach, became the

first blind parliamentarian of Europe and an eminent states-
man in Belgium; and the other, Alexandre Fournier, became
famous for his phenomenal skill as a finger reader, which he
demonstrated in many countries. In 1806, when Haüy was
invited by the Tsar of Russia to come to that country to start
a school for the blind, he took his wife and Fournier with
him.

Haüy started to Russia by way of Germany. In Berlin, his
fame had preceded him and he was invited to speak before
the Academy of Sciences. The learned members were so impressed that they arranged for a demonstration before King
Friederich Wilhelm III and Queen Louise of Prussia. The
King, in turn, was so moved that he asked Haüy to remain in
Germany long enough to set up a school there. Haüy drew up
the plans, selected Dr. August Zeune, a distinguished geogra-
pher, to head the new venture, and witnessed its inauguration
in Steglitz, near Berlin, in August 1806. This soon became
one of the leading schools for the blind in Europe.

Continuing on his way to Russia, Haüy passed through
Vienna, where he found that a school had already been started
in 1804 by Johann Wilhelm Klein, a former district director
for the poor. Recognizing lack of education as a cause of
poverty among the blind, he resolved to open a school for
blind children. Like Haüy, Klein began with one pupil, a
blind boy named Jacob Braun. Through many experiments,.
Klein developed a sound educational program which reflected the influence of Maria von Paradis, whose home was
in Vienna, and avoided the charitable aspects to which Haüy
had succumbed. Klein was competent in all that he did and
soon commanded royal support for his school. He studied the
problems of the education of the blind and the application of
sound pedagogy to them.

The interest of this competent educator reached out to
blind children whom he could not bring within his school,
and he made perhaps the earliest attempts to have them accepted in schools for the seeing. Klein gave early thought to
the question of securing able teachers and produced a *Teacher's Manual for the Education of the Blind.* Under Klein's

leadership, extending through fifty years, the Vienna School became outstanding and continued its good work until the Hitler regime, when the school buildings were used as a home for the aged. The library, with the world's finest collection of books on the blind, was destroyed in World War II.

When Haüy finally reached Russia, he was given a cold reception and was assured by officials that Russia had no blind. Despite his invitation from the Tsar, Haüy waited several years before he was allowed to see him. In the meantime, he secured some help from the mother Tsarina which enabled him to assemble a few blind children, but language difficulties and lack of equipment made it more of an asylum than a school.

Haüy returned to Paris in 1817, wearing a decoration of the Order of St. Vladimir given him by the Tsar. Discouraged and embittered by the turn of events in his own school, he died on March 19, 1822, at the age of seventy-seven. "The finest tribute to Haüy's memory," writes Ishbel Ross, "was the string of schools modelled after his that by this time dotted Europe." [7] In 1861, the French government unveiled a marble bust of Haüy in one of the courts of the school he had founded.

The tragic end of Valentin Haüy is not hard to understand, considering the social forces prevailing at the time, the abyss of ignorance about the blind, and the illiteracy of the blind themselves. And while positive credit must be given to him for the practical development of an embossed type and as the first to accept the challenge of Rousseau to apply the metaphysics of the earlier philosophers to the education of the blind, it must be acknowledged that he did little to ameliorate their condition.

Valentin Haüy was not a sound educator nor a good psychologist in his dealings with people. His mistakes were fundamental. His theory that the style of a type to be read by touch must also be pleasing to the eye and his determination "to preserve the strictest analogy between the means of educating the blind and the sighted" were fallacies that made deep impressions on later educators. It is obvious that the success of Haüy's exhibitions went to his head and that much of his educational procedure was based on making them successful rather than on training the young blind to succeed in fields that would provide a living and enable them to find suitable positions in society. And yet Samuel Gridley Howe, who was most critical of his shows and parades, could write in 1833: "Haüy merits the endearing title 'father of the blind'; a reward richer than a crown; a title more truly glorious than that of conqueror." [8]

3 STIRRINGS IN
EUROPE

ABOUT the same time that Haüy opened the first school in Paris, there were stirrings of concern for blind children in the British Isles. The first practical attempt to alleviate the condition of the sightless in England began in Liverpool under the leadership of Edward Rushton, who had served as mate on a slave ship. On what proved to be his last voyage, all of the miserable negroes in the hold were attacked by a malignant ophthalmia. The kindly mate was so distressed that he went among them to help them and in this way contracted the disease, which seriously impaired his sight.

Obliged to give up the sea, Rushton settled in Liverpool and became engaged in many charitable ventures. He proceeded to enlist the support of others, and a School for the Indigent Blind was opened in 1791. It was hardly a school, since no literary studies were taught. Its object was to teach poor visually handicapped children to work at trades, to sing in churches, and to play the organ. Incidentally, it may be mentioned that, after thirty-three years of blindness, Rushton's sight was restored through an operation in 1807.

As early as 1744, there had been some interest in educating the blind in Scotland, for in that year there appeared in the *Edinburgh Magazine and Review* a proposed system of education for the sightless. This, however, had no immediate result. Later, the Scots were moved by a vigorous living example of what an educated blind person could accomplish.

Thomas Blacklock, blinded at the age of six months, had become a distinguished preacher and theologian and a fluent writer of verse. In 1783, he wrote an article on "The Blind" for the *Encyclopaedia Britannica,* then published in Edinburgh.

Blacklock made a translation of the *Essay on the Education of the Blind* written by Haüy in 1786, which was not published until two years after his death in 1791. Before his death, however, Blacklock had discussed the establishment of a school for the blind with Mr. David Miller, an excellent teacher who, like Blacklock, had been blind from early childhood. Miller enlisted the aid of the Rev. David Johnson, and together they established in 1793 the Edinburgh Blind Asylum with nine pupils. Its object was "to render the blind happy in themselves and useful to society."

At Bristol, England, in the same year, an Asylum and Industrial School for the Blind was opened by two members of the Society of Friends, with four boys and two girls as pupils. At first, the pupils came to the school daily, but in 1803 residential accommodations were provided and later a shop for employment was added, despite the original objective "not to employ the blind after education, but to teach them the means of getting a living by work." This objective struck a sound note which, unfortunately, was not followed out by the succeeding English institutions, most of which have workshops attached to them into which pupils are automatically transferred when schooling terminates. The fourth British school to be founded in the eighteenth century was the School for the Indigent Blind at St. George's, Southwark, in 1799. Here the pupils were to be "educated, maintained, and taught a trade."

In the early years of the nineteenth century, schools for the blind sprang up in many European countries. Many of them were included in the string of schools that dot Europe and stand as a tribute to Valentin Haüy. Others, however, were outside the orbit of Haüy and must be attributed to the social influences of the time, such as Klein's School in Vienna, which became one of the soundest schools educationally, and the English schools motivated largely by the desire to teach blind children trades in order to enable them to work. Before Haüy, the father of the education of the blind, died in 1822, the following schools were established:

1804   Austria at Vienna, by Dr. Johann Wilhelm Klein;

1806   Germany at Steglitz, near Berlin, by August Zeune;

1807   Italy at Milan, by Cav. Michele Barozzi;

1808   Holland at Amsterdam, by an association of Free Masons;

        Bohemia at Prague, by a charitable society;

        Sweden at Stockholm, by Per Aron Borg;

1809   Russia at St. Petersburg, by Valentin Haüy;

        Switzerland at Zurich, by Dr. Hirzel;

1810   Ireland at Dublin, by Protestants;

1811   Denmark at Copenhagen, by the "Society of the Chain" (Masons) ;

1812   Scotland at Aberdeen, "through the munificence of Miss Cruikshank";

1815   Ireland at Dublin, by Roman Catholics;

1816   Belgium at Brussels, by Canonicus Triest;

1818   Italy at Naples, by Dominique Martuscelli;

1820   Spain at Barcelona, by M. Richard.

While it is apparent that all of these early schools differed widely in their methods and somewhat in their objectives, they had in common the desire to alleviate the lot of the blind by beginning with children. To analyze their motives or to appraise their achievements would avail little, but it may be of interest to have an evaluation of these projects from the pen of a competent person interested in this form of welfare and earnestly seeking ways to help blind children. In 1830, Samuel Gridley Howe, about to open the first school for the blind to be chartered in America, went to Europe to learn their ways.

Howe visited most of the schools in Europe, omitting unfortunately the one in Vienna where he would have learned the most, and submitted to his trustees his reactions to their methods. He had a good word for the German institutions except the one at Berlin. There he considered Dr. Zeune a capable leader who was handicapped in his choice of teachers by government interference, a fact which made Howe prefer schools under voluntary auspices.

The institution for the Education of the Blind in Paris [Howe reported], as it is the oldest, and as there is about it more of a show and parade than any other in Europe, has also the reputation of being the best; but if one judges the tree by its fruits, and not by its flowers and foliage, this will not be his conclusion.

Its founder and the great benefactor of the blind, the Abbé Haüy, invented and put into practice many contrivances for the education of the blind; and otherwise rendered the institution excellent for the age, and the time it had existed; but as he left it, so has it since remained. . . .

The great fault of the Parisian Institution is the diversity of employment to which the pupils are put; and the effort made to enable them to perform surprising but useless tricks. The same degree of intellectual education is given to all, without reference to destination in life; and a poor boy who is to get his livelihood by weaving or whip-making is as well instructed in mathematics and polite literature as he who is to pursue a literary career.

Of all the British schools, Dr. Howe was most impressed by the one in Edinburgh which he considered

on the whole, the best I saw in Europe; it comes nearer than any other to the attainment of the great object of blind schools; viz., enabling the pupils to support themselves by their own efforts in after life. The establishment is not so showy as that in Paris, nor has it the same means which the latter possesses, and which receives an allowance of 60,000 francs, or $12,000 per annum from the government; nor has it printed books for their use; still they receive most excellent education and learn some useful trades.[1]

The acid test to which Dr. Howe put education was whether or not it qualified blind boys and girls to attain "the great object of blind schools; viz., enabling the pupils to support themselves by their own efforts in after life." Or, as the objective of the Bristol School stated, "not to employ the blind after being educated, but to teach them the means of getting a living by work." It is perhaps not unfair to say that few schools in Europe have every fully attained that objective.

The seeing world, however, may be blamed for this situation, for it was not then, nor is it now, ready to accept the blind as fully employable. But at that early time, few efforts were made in that direction or in developing methods of placement. It seemed easier to attach hostels and workshops to the schools and thus provide for the after care of the students. This set the pattern still common in Europe: school attendance beginning at the age of five to eight and continuing for seven to ten years, then the shop. Of course, a few able students rise above this and go on to higher education. But too few find useful places in the social and economic world.

An interesting attempt to improve that situation in England was made by Thomas Rhodes Armitage, who, in 1868, brought together in one organization the many groups interested in the blind under the name of the British and Foreign Blind Association, now known as the Royal National Institute for the Blind. Dr. Armitage, a successful physician who had to give up his practice at the age of thirty-six because of failing sight, turned his attention to those who were similarly handicapped. He became gravely concerned over the fact that the schools for blind youth were not integrating their graduates into society. He had been to the Paris School, where, under the able leadership of Dr. Sebastien Guillié (a successor of Valentin Haüy), its graduates were so well trained as teachers of music, organists, and piano tuners that 30 per cent were able to earn their own living; whereas in England, Dr. Armitage found that not 1 per cent were able to do this.

Dr. Armitage was resolved that England should do better. He tried to persuade some of the English schools to develop new methods and even offered to pay all of the expenses of the experiments. Just at this time, Francis J. Campbell happened to call on Dr. Armitage and through him the latter found further support for his convictions. Mr. Campbell was the blind head of the music department at Perkins Institution, where he had demonstrated the practical advantages of a superior musical education. Of twenty pupils whom he had trained there, nineteen were supporting themselves. Because of the ill health of his wife, Campbell had brought her to Europe and had spent a year studying music in Leipzig. He was on his way home when he met and talked with Dr. Armitage.

After again trying in vain to get one of the older institutions to make its objective the placement of its graduates, Dr. Armitage decided to open a new school. He persuaded Mr. Campbell to change his plans and to remain in England. Together they opened in 1872 the Royal Normal College and Academy of Music with two pupils, both from the town of Leeds. "Mr. C.," wrote Dr. Howe in his Perkins report for 1874,

could not find suitably trained teachers in London; and sought some who had been trained in our school. He applied to me to give leave of absence to one of our teachers to help him, and I consented with pleasure. He then applied for another and another as his school grew; and he obtained them because I felt bound by duty to the cause to help what was in reality an American institution, struggling for existence in a foreign land, which would give the blind greater advantages than any existing there . . . The college is, however, an exotic, and it will require the most skillful care and attention by persons of pure and high motives to make it take firm root and attain large growth in its foreign soil.[2]

This type of leadership was generously given by the Campbell family, for the founder was succeeded first by his son Guy and then by his son's widow. Glasgow University awarded the honorary degree of LL.D. to the founder of the Royal Normal College, and in 1909 he became Sir Francis Campbell in recognition of what he had done to give the blind of England the benefits of new ways of finding a rightful place in life. After his death on December 28, 1935, Sir Francis' body was returned to America and buried in the family plot at South Acton, Massachusetts, under a tombstone inscribed: "His life work was for those who, like himself, were bereft of sight. And he left an example of noble courage and untiring zeal that will ever be an inspiration to the blind."

Under the Campbell leadership, the Royal Normal College provided promising blind youth with superior training in music. But it did more. Sir Francis traveled throughout the country, placing his organists in village churches and seeking work for his highly trained piano tuners. The School also trained blind youth in the practical arts, including typing and shorthand, and soon many graduates of this department were finding employment in the business world. In 1885, the College had 170 students, and it is reported that 80 per cent of its graduates were entirely self-supporting, proving the point made by Dr. Armitage. But it took methods and efforts not then, nor even now, found in many English schools. It was not until World War II that the British could report as many blind persons working in open industry as they had in sheltered shops.

England has two other schools for secondary education that are outstanding. They do not offer definite terminal vocational courses as the Royal Normal College does, for they are preparatory schools leading to the universities. The first and older is Worcester College, founded in 1889, and established along the lines of the public schools for seeing boys. It was planned originally as "a school for the blind sons of gentlemen," and in its earliest years this described its clientele. It is only in very recent years that the College has accepted qualified boys from the common elementary schools. Not until 1921 was similar provision made to prepare promising girls for matriculation into the universities. In that year, Chorleywood College was opened by the National Institute for the Blind. Both of these schools prepare promising youth for higher education, and in this they have had an excellent record, owing perhaps to careful selection, since their total enrollment is only about 120. This is about $12\frac{1}{2}$ per cent of the number of pupils in schools for the blind and about the same percentage as of seeing boys and girls who go on to higher education in that country.

Another school of this type is the one at Marburg an der Lahn, Germany, founded in 1916, where in 1952 there were fifty-one students. One-half of these are war-blinded; the other half have come up through the schools for the blind. Because of the great care in selection, the percentage of blind students going to college in Germany is smaller than the percentage of seeing boys and girls.

As it is not possible to give space to a historical report of all the educational provisions for the blind in England or to treat fully the development in other countries, it may be well to review the present facilities for the education of blind children as reported at the International Conference of Educators of Blind Youth held at Bussum, Holland, in July 1952.[3] This summary does not include the facilities in the United States or those behind the Iron Curtain. Conditions in this country will be discussed later and a report on the facilities in Russia and its satellites will have to be delayed until more information is available. At Bussum, Yugoslavia was represented by a capable delegation who made a good report of their six elementary schools with 275 pupils and 75 teachers and of three special schools with about 100 students. The three special schools, however, were the product of the preceding regime.

Thirty-four nations sent delegates to Bussum, making it the most widely representative conference on the blind ever held. Included in the published report of the conference are summaries of the educational facilities for blind children in most of the countries represented. Much of this material came originally from a survey of blind children made for the United Nations in December 1950.[4] This was supplemented by reports from other countries represented at Bussum where all reports were checked and amplified by the respective delegations before publication in the conference report.

Twenty-eight countries outside of the United States reported a total of 354 schools, with an enrollment of about 20,000 pupils. Figures compiled in 1953 by Dr. Guy Dingemans of Paris, after a study of facilities for handicapped children in Latin America, make it possible to add to these figures 34 more schools for blind children in that area, with an enrollment of less than 2,000. To complete the record, the 57 schools in the United States with enrollments in that year totaling 6,909 should be added. For most of the free world, this makes a grand total of approximately 450 schools giving instruction to nearly 30,000 children—not a very impressive impact on the number of blind children in the world, which must total at least two million.

According to the reports submitted at Bussum, Japan had the largest number of schools—74, enrolling 4,855 pupils in

1950—while the United States reported the largest number of pupils—6,909 in 57 schools. France has 30 schools, 4 national and 26 provincial, none offering instruction beyond the elementary level. England and Wales together have 19 elementary schools and 3 at the secondary level. Italy has one of the most comprehensive schemes with 18 elementary schools, each with a kindergarten; 12 professional schools, established in 1949; and 2 technical high schools and a program for teacher training. At the Institute of Bologna, a boarding house is maintained for blind students attending the university.

Practically all of these institutions are residential, modeled after the first school of Valentin Haüy, or are developments from what were originally asylums. Nearly all of the European and many other schools outside of North America follow the pattern laid down by Napoleon in 1800, that blind children be admitted at the age of seven and remain under instruction for eight years. There are some variations in this, a few accepting children at five (including all in England) and several continuing their stay for ten years. All of this is based on chronological age and has little relation to the child's mental age or academic achievement. Recently, provision has been made for pupils to continue beyond the legal maximum age for from two to five years at vocational studies. Only England, Germany, Italy, Sweden, and Yugoslavia report special secondary schools. There is some provision, however, for exceptional students to secure the equivalent of our high-school courses by attending schools for the seeing.

Educators of the blind are becoming aware of the shortcomings of such a stereotyped schedule and of the need for more flexible provisions to match the individual aptitudes of blind children. This led to the inclusion in the Bussum program of a session on "The Needs of the Blind Child for Continued Elementary Education." Its conclusions are summed up in the resolution which stated in part:

The Conference feels that in countries where formal education terminates at a fixed age, there should be an opportunity for continued training in general education which will provide cultural development as well as industrial skills . . . The objective of all countries should be to train blind boys and girls to be able to take their places in the economic and social life of the communities in which they live . . . The Conference feels that schools for the blind should continue their general education program to a point where their graduates are equipped to attain that objective . . . The Conference feels that it is the responsibility of schools to train their youth to this way of life and that their responsibility is not over at a specified age when transfer is made to the sheltered shop. Emancipation from this pattern is being increasingly provided for the gifted . . . It must be expanded to include all blind youth capable of earning their way in the humbler walks of life.[5]

Further study of the Bussum report reveals the voids that exist in the prevailing program for the years before entering school and after leaving. For the preschool years, only a few countries have any definite programs and among them there is a wide difference of methods. In the United States, educators of the blind feel that the young child should be retained in the home, if at all possible, so that there are only two residential nursery schools and five day schools for this age group.

In England, while educators admit that the home is the proper place for the young blind child, there is a strong feeling that no home is adequate to cope with the situation; so they have seven nursery schools, called Sunshine Homes, and every encouragement is given to parents to send their children to them. Many countries, in increasing numbers, are showing interest in a program for these formative years, and several delegates reported plans for having teachers or social workers visit in the homes, while booklets of guidance and help have been made available for distribution to parents.

Looking toward the after-school days, there is little well-planned and organized activity leading to placement in open industry beyond the relatively small number that complete higher education, and even these are largely left to shift for themselves. Practically no schools outside of the United States take any responsibility for after-school placement in work situations. Some depend on the government labor offices, but most look to the voluntary blind societies to help young people when they leave school. This also applies to guidance programs. Several schools stated that the teachers who know the pupils best can best advise them.

The same attitude prevails toward psychological and achievement tests. One country reported "no tests are performed, as the opinion prevails that the educators teaching and watching the pupils for some years can give the necessary hints for the choice of vocations." In England, psychological tests are not yet widely used, but Scotland reports using all that are available. Switzerland has its blind children tested in the psychometric clinics for seeing children. Canada uses tests "in some schools" and Austria reports using them "now and again." Countries using modern tests—and this usually means those developed at Perkins Institution under Dr. Samuel P. Hayes—include Finland, Japan, New Zealand, Norway, and Sweden.

Perhaps the best way to sum up the aspirations that all countries have for the education of their blind children is to quote from the resolution adopted by the Conference of Workers for the Blind held at Merton College, Oxford, in August 1949, where the committee to plan for the Bussum Conference was organized. The Oxford Conference went on record as follows:

To enable blind persons to participate fully in the life of the community and to contribute to its strength, blind persons, whether children, young persons, or adults, should be given full opportunity for general and vocational education, in schools adequately equipped for the education of the blind, and with fully qualified teachers.

The Conference puts on record its conviction that every national system of education should ensure to all blind children education according to their interests and aptitudes, at least equal to that which they would have received if they had not been blind.[6]

4 PIONEERING IN AMERICA

THE impetus to educate the blind in the United States did not come in the spectacular way that impelled Valentin Haüy to devote his life to the sightless after beholding the burlesque of the blind musicians at the Café Saint Ovide. But there is a certain drama in the chance way in which those interested in the blind happened to find the man who was to become the Haüy of America. On an afternoon in the summer of 1831, a group of Boston men were walking down Boylston Street discussing how the asylum for the blind incorporated by the Legislature in 1829 could be gotten under way.

As they walked, Dr. John D. Fisher, who had originated the idea, looked up and saw a dashing young man approaching. Turning to the others, he said: "Here is Howe, the very man we have been looking for all the time." [1] "The very man" was Samuel Gridley Howe, recently returned from participation in the Greek struggle for freedom and looking for new fields to conquer. Approached on the matter, young Howe eagerly accepted, on the condition that he might first go to Europe to study the methods in use over there, which were attracting world-wide attention.

Howe did not have the background of interest that had impelled Valentin Haüy into this field of humanitarian work. He had not met Maria von Paradis, nor had he heard of the blind man of Puiseau. He had not participated in the discussions of such men as Voltaire, Rousseau, and Diderot, who had done so much to mold the social thinking of pre-Revolutionary France. But Howe did have some of that humanitarian philosophy which was beginning to sweep over the world. In no place did it find more fertile soil than in Boston. So it was in 1826, when Dr. John D. Fisher returned from medical studies in France and told of what was being done for the blind at the Haüy school and the need for similar efforts in this country. A sympathetic response immediately arose from all sides of Beacon Hill and, indeed, from the summit of the Hill itself, for none were more eager to help than the legislators assembled in the State House. Encouraged by this response, Dr. Fisher called a meeting on February 10, 1829, in the Exchange Coffee House in Boston, where he gave an account of the work that he had observed in Europe. Supported by correspondence with Robert Johnston, then head of the school in Edinburgh, Fisher pointed out that the time was ripe for similar help for blind children in this country.

As the Legislature was then in session, many members of the General Court attended the meeting and were moved by Dr. Fisher's plea. When the incorporators whom Dr. Fisher had gathered about him made application for a charter, the members of the Court were quick to grant it. On March 2, 1829, an Act of Incorporation created the New-England Asylum for the Blind for the purpose of educating blind persons, and six weeks later a recess commission was appointed to make a study of the blind within the Commonwealth. At the end of a year, a board of twelve trustees was appointed and officers were elected. Another year elapsed before the fateful meeting on Boylston Street and the finding of "the very man."

In the enabling legislation that created the New-England Asylum for the Blind appears a list of the names of the incorporators. This is headed by Jonathan Phillips, who had been elected president, and immediately following is the name William Prescott. The fact that this name is so high on the list supports a feeling that is soon developed in reading the early records that here is a man whose contribution to the new institution must have been great. And so it was, for William Hickling Prescott, born in Boston on May 4, 1796, could contribute more than the others because he himself lived in a darkened world. Despite his visual handicap, Prescott became a historian whose works to this day are still considered standard both for historical acumen and for scholarly writing. But his place among the great of the blind world has not always been as widely acknowledged and his part in the founding of the pioneer school has certainly not been sufficiently acclaimed.

While preparing for the writing of *Ferdinand and Isabella,* his first book, which took ten years to write, Prescott published a number of articles in the *North American Review.* Among these was one in the July 1830 issue which told of the legislation creating the new asylum for the blind. Its contents reveal a wide knowledge of the plight of the sightless and of work for their benefit. Such a study could only come from a competent student of that field and the article is certainly the equal of many of the famed "letters on the blind" that were appearing at the time. Some parts of the article, George Ticknor, his biographer, wrote, "are so obviously the result of his own experience, that they should be remembered as expressions of his personal character." [2]

Samuel Gridley Howe, "the very man" who was to put life into the newly chartered asylum for the blind, was born on November 10, 1801, the second of three sons brought up in the comfortable, spacious home of a well-to-do Boston family. His father, a dealer in naval supplies and a maker of cordage, sold to the government during the War of 1812 large quantities of naval supplies for which he was never fully paid. This left the family in such straitened circumstances that only one of the three sons could be sent to college. The father made his choice by having all three boys read passages from the Scriptures, and as Sam read better than the others, he was selected.

Howe was entered in Brown University rather than Harvard because its political affiliations were more in line with his father's thinking than was the university in Cambridge. Here he was not as outstanding in his studies as in his pranks. He succeeded, however, in graduating in 1821 at the age of twenty. Returning to Boston, Howe attended lectures at the Harvard Medical School and clinics at the Massachusetts General Hospital. He proved to be a most promising student, and his instructors predicted a great career in medicine.

> Suddenly he astounded them and the Boston community [Dr. James G. Mumford relates] by announcing that he was going to Greece. Even the restrained writers of the day flutter with protest and amazement when they tell of it . . . The young man was called Byron-mad. No one encouraged him except one eminent man, Gilbert Stuart, the artist, now growing old, who faltered that his heart also was in the venture, if only the times were still young for him. He helped Howe to go. He gave him money, got for him a letter from Edward Everett to an old friend in Greece, and with a quavering blessing sent him on his way.[3]

There are other interpretations of young Howe's desire to go to Greece. Many feel that he was caught up in that surge to help the underprivileged that was sweeping over America at the time; and others attribute it to a desire to escape from an unrequited love affair, for which theory there is considerable evidence. Whatever may have been the reason that impelled the young physician to leave Boston and a promising medical career, he sailed for Greece in November of 1824.

The practical way in which Howe administered projects of relief to the distressed folk of that country brought out the traits that were to make him a great social reformer. In these undertakings he was assisted by Dr. John Dennison Russ, who later was to open the school for the blind in New York; Dr. Edward Jarvis, afterward associated with Dr. Howe at Perkins; and George Finlay, who became the historian of Greece. While engaged in this work, Howe contracted "swamp fever," which made it necessary for him to leave Greece.

From January 30, 1830, until July of that year, there is no entry in his Journal, but it is known that he turned westward and, seeking recuperation, journeyed slowly through Switzerland and Italy until he reached Paris. There he planned to study surgery, but instead he went to England, where he remained ten weeks, and then to Boston, arriving April 16,

1831. It was at this crucial time that Howe met the little group of men, and Dr. Fisher, seeing the young hero from Greece, declared him to be "the very man."

On August 18, 1831, Samuel Gridley Howe was appointed director of the already incorporated New-England Asylum for the Blind. Before undertaking its implementation, it was agreed that the new Director should go to Europe to observe the work there and to engage necessary teachers. Howe visited several schools for the blind on the Continent, but missed the best one, at Vienna. He also went to those in Scotland and England and was most favorably impressed with the school at Edinburgh. His impressions of these visits have already been quoted in the evaluation of the early work in Europe. A brief summary of his reactions is found in his statement that the schools which he saw were "beacons to warn rather than lights to guide."

His visits to the European schools, however, did produce some positive convictions that were to guide Howe as he organized the school for the blind in Boston. These were:

1. That each blind child must be considered as an individual and be trained in accordance with his personal ability and opportunity to use the training in his community.

2. That the curriculum of a school for the blind should be well rounded and conform insofar as possible to that of the common schools, but that more music and crafts should be provided.

3. That the main objective must be to train blind youth to be able to take their places in the social and economic life of their home communities as contributing members.

With these principles in mind, Howe set out to find pupils for the new undertaking.

In the year 1832 [he wrote], while inquiring for blind children suitable for instruction in our project, I heard of a family in Andover in which there were several such, and immediately drove out thither with my friend and co-worker, Dr. John D. Fisher. As we approached the toll house, and halted to pay the toll, I saw by the roadside two pretty little girls, one about six, the other about eight years old, tidily dressed, and standing hand in hand hard by the toll house . . . On looking more closely, I saw that they were both totally blind. It was a touching and interesting scene.[4]

Abby and Sophia Carter became Dr. Howe's first pupils and later his joy and pride, for they accompanied him on many demonstration trips. Although keeping in contact with their family, the two girls continued to live at the Institution throughout their lives. Abby died in 1875 and Sophia in 1888.

Four other children were found, and in August 1832 the little school began with Dr. Howe as director and two teachers, M. Trenchéri, a literary teacher from the Paris School, and John Pringle of the Edinburgh School as teacher of crafts. Housing the new school presented problems. The first sessions were held in Howe's family home. The father, now elderly, seemed not to object and the Howe sisters living at home entered joyfully into the enterprise. But this arrangement had shortcomings in addition to lack of space when the numbers multiplied to twenty.

At this juncture, Colonel Thomas H. Perkins stepped into the breach, offering to give his spacious mansion and gardens, occupying a quarter acre of land, as a permanent home for the blind school, provided the citizens of Boston raised $50,000 for its support. By this time, the blind asylum was fast becoming the favorite charity of Boston. The state increased its appropriation and fairs were held by the first ladies of this benevolent city. A special fair brought in $11,000, Jonathan Phillips gave $5,000, while the director (taking his six blind pupils) "went about the state and about New England with them, giving exhibitions and raising money." The $50,000 was secured within a month and the school moved into the big house on Pearl Street.

The school continued to expand and in 1837 more space was needed. A great hotel built on the heights of South Boston overlooking the harbor and Dorchester Bay had failed in the financial depression of that year and came on the market. Here was the ideal site for the school, but before it could be purchased consent had to be secured from Colonel Perkins to sell the Pearl Street house, for a condition of the gift had been that it must be used for the blind or revert to him or to his heirs. Colonel Perkins proved generous and authorized the sale of his house. In 1839 the school moved into the hotel, where it remained until 1912. In that year, the Institution, with its older pupils, moved to the present site in Watertown, and in the following year the Kindergarten, which had been opened in Jamaica Plain in 1886, joined it.

In gratitude to Colonel Perkins, the trustees named the growing enterprise Perkins Institution and Massachusetts Asylum for the Blind. This was changed again in 1877 when the word "School" replaced the term "Asylum." And in November 1955, the name was again changed by vote of the Corporation and the Trustees, to "Perkins School for the Blind," in order to eliminate the present implications of the word "Institution," with which a former generation replaced "Asylum." The far-sighted Dr. Howe was not unmindful of the need for change, for in 1874 he wrote:

For these, and other like causes, I desire and advise that the name of our Institution be made shorter and simpler: and that it may more clearly define its nature and its objects, the best title which occurs to me is that of *New England School for the Blind*. But, if the heirs of Mr. Perkins should feel aggrieved by the substitution of another name for his, then call it *Perkins School for the Blind*. The simpler and more appropriate name will probably be adopted when there shall be none to object or to feel aggrieved.[5]

Attaching and continuing the name of Perkins has seemed strange to many for beyond the gift of his house and the assent to its sale and his personal service for a few years on the Board of Trustees, Colonel Perkins knew little of and did little for the blind. But he was one of the great tycoons of his day in the commerce of ships which plied from the Port of Boston to all parts of the world. It is said that when asked by George Washington to be Secretary of the Navy, he declined, stating that he owned and operated more ships than the United States Government.

It is truly the irony of fame that the school for the blind, which was in large measure the creation of Samuel Gridley Howe, does not bear his name except as casually applied to the main building of the Watertown plant, and there is a double irony in the fact that the school for idiots which he also founded and directed for twenty-five years is now the Walter E. Fernald School for the Feeble-Minded, with the Howe name attached only to an auditorium at the present site in Waverley. Nevertheless, the fame of Samuel Gridley Howe is secure among those who know of his prowess and his pioneering. And he himself would probably have preferred to have his memory kept alive in good works that he initiated rather than see it inscribed on walls of brick and mortar. And, asked John Greenleaf Whittier, in his poem, "The Hero":

> Wouldst know him now? Behold him,
> The Cadmus of the blind,
> Giving the dumb lip language,
> The idiot clay a mind.

And as Oliver Wendell Holmes wrote in his Memorial Tribute:

> He touched the eyelids of the blind,
> And lo! the veil withdrawn,
> As o'er the midnight of the mind
> He led the light of dawn.

Students of the welfare of the blind will continue to recognize Howe as the first to set forth the high principle that, through education and training, those with impaired vision could and should contribute to the society in which they live. But that is only a small segment of the wide interests of this indomitable man. His fertile mind and potent hand were manifest in all of the important movements of his time; often, however, behind the scenes, as in the common-school movement with Horace Mann in the forefront; the crusade for the insane with Dorothea Dix leading; the antislavery movement which led him to support John Brown and after the Harper's Ferry raid to go to Canada fearing arrest. Howe gave equal impetus to the opening of a school that would teach the mute to speak. This led to the creation of what is now the Clarke School for the Deaf in Northampton. For a time, Howe served in the Massachusetts Legislature, and while there he introduced the resolution that led to the investigation and modernization of prisons.

Howe, wrote Dr. Mumford, had "an eager and inquiring soul, looking ever for something new, always appearing to tilt at windmills and not content to tread in beaten paths, or gather laurels in familiar fields." [6] This undoubtedly explains his great absorption in Laura Bridgman as soon as he had the new school operating, a project that brought him universal fame and thus led to many trips abroad where he was hailed with adulation—"soft soap," he called it in his letters to friends.

When the Civil War broke out, Dr. Howe was asked to make a survey of the sanitary conditions of the Massachusetts troops in the field at and around Washington. This meant many trips to Washington. Perhaps the most notable outcome of this activity was when he took his wife with him and she, inspired by the watch fires in the night, the faces of marching men and their singing voices, wrote with a stub of pencil on a scrap of Sanitary Commission paper "The Battle Hymn of the Republic." And so, wrote Dr. Mumford, "to the average American of today, Samuel Howe is known, if at all, as the half-forgotten husband only of that distinguished veteran poetess, Julia Ward Howe. Truly the pen is mightier than the sword." [7]

Samuel Gridley Howe and John D. Fisher were not lone voices crying in the wilderness for the amelioration of the lot of the blind. Almost simultaneously, voices were being raised in New York and Philadelphia. In New York, William Wood, a benevolent bookseller, became concerned about the neglect of blind children in that city. He solicited the interest of Dr. Samuel Akerly, a leader in the education of the deaf, and "a petition was prepared and presented to the legislature in 1831; on April 21 of that year, a society was incorporated under the title of the New-York Institution for the Blind." [8]

In the summer of 1831, and quite independently, Dr. John Dennison Russ, a former associate of Dr. Howe as almoner of relief in Greece, became interested in blind boys whom he had observed in the city almshouse, and resolved to do something about them. Learning of Dr. Russ's plans, the president of the new society invited Russ to coöperate with them and to become a member of its board. This he did and in February 1832, when it was decided to take the boys from the almshouse and begin their instruction, Dr. Russ volunteered to be the first teacher. A room was rented in a house on Canal Street and work began on March 15, 1832. This was done "with a view to exhibitions, after attaining proficiency, so that interest might be excited in the objects of the association."

Apparently the venture into the education of the blind in New York had trouble in getting under way, for the report of the Institution for 1841 stated "that it was a matter of some difficulty to find among our intelligent and benevolent citizens twenty gentlemen who were willing to be appointed to its first Board of Managers." And in 1845, its purpose was still not clear to some, while "others assumed that it was an Asylum for the indigent blind, erected for the purpose of testing by actual experiment the lowest possible sum upon which its subjects could be fed and clothed." [9]

The New York Institute's great day came later when in 1863 William Bell Wait took charge, at the age of twenty-four. During his thirty-eight years at the school, Wait became a potent factor in the field of the blind. Trained as a lawyer, he made careful surveys of existing conditions and, after assembling the facts, used his findings in the formulating of his programs. One of his first resolves was to strengthen the academic instruction at the expense of craft training.

But it was not until 1890 that he made the legal changes that represented his convictions on educational policy. In that year, supervision of the school was transferred from the Department of Welfare to the Department of Education, thereby removing the stigma of pauperism that the former connection implied. The name was changed to the New York Institute for the Education of the Blind and Wait's own title from Superintendent to Principal. The curriculum became the same as that followed by the State Board of Education and blind pupils took the Board of Regents' examinations given to all public-school children.

New York had its counterpart of Colonel Perkins in the wealthy merchant, James Boorman, who in 1837 gave to the school his mansion and land equivalent to a city block, known as Strawberry Hill, then out in the country, but now located at the corner of 9th Avenue and 34th Street. The school is proud of the fact that for a time one of its teachers was Grover Cleveland, later president of the United States. It takes pride also in its most distinguished pupil, Fanny Crosby, the famous blind hymn writer, many of whose works enliven the Moody and Sankey *Hymnal*.

After completing her studies, Fanny Crosby remained at the school and for twenty-three years taught grammar and history. The friend of three presidents, Tyler, Polk, and Cleveland, Miss Crosby attracted many distinguished visitors to Strawberry Hill. Interesting stories are told of the blind hymnist. It is said that she liked to sleep "in a bed of roses" and that on all of her travels she always carried a small American flag. She died in Bridgeport, Connecticut, in 1915 at the age of ninety-five. The school remained at Strawberry Hill until 1924 when, under the strong and understanding leadership of Dr. Edward M. Van Cleve, it was moved to its present beautiful location on Pelham Parkway.

As early as 1824, interest in the blind was expressed in Philadelphia among the Quakers. Once again, provision for the education of the deaf stimulated interest in the blind. A member of the Society of Friends, Robert Vaux, mentioned the matter to Joshua Francis Fisher, who, in 1830, went to Europe to study the methods employed in schools there. Shortly after his return in the autumn of 1832, Julius R. Friedlander, a German, who had observed schools for the blind in Berlin, London, and Paris, arrived in Philadelphia

with the intention of starting a school. He carried with him
letters to two members of the Society of Friends, one of whom
was Robert Vaux.

This fortuitous circumstance enabled the work for the
blind in Philadelphia to get a good start under experienced
leadership. Friedlander immediately was given an opportunity to teach a small group of blind boys. On January 21,
1833, a meeting was called to consider organization. On
March 5, 1833, officers were elected and Friedlander was appointed as principal. The Act of Incorporation was approved
on January 27, 1834, officially creating the Pennsylvania Institution for the Instruction of the Blind.

In the school's formative days, Friedlander's chief contribution came through his interest in embossed books. The
first book embossed for the blind in America was produced
at the Philadelphia school. Friedlander is credited with having invented a form of line type and he took an active part in
the search for a satisfactory type. He did not remain long
as head of the Philadelphia school, for, failing in health,
he had to give up his work. He died in Philadelphia on
March 17, 1838.

After a succession of superintendents, Edward E. Allen, a
teacher at Perkins and prior to that at the Royal Normal College in London, took charge in 1890 and in 1899 moved the
school from downtown Philadelphia to a new site with large
grounds in Overbrook, just over the city line. Here under
Allen's direction the impressive structure in Spanish archi-
tectural style was erected where it now stands amid lovely
gardens.

This was the beginning of the exodus of schools for the
blind from the cities to garden suburbs that took place in
the early part of the century. In 1913, Allen moved Perkins
from South Boston to Watertown and in 1924, Van Cleve
built the New York school at its present location. During
those years, the leaders of the schools in Boston, New York,
and Philadelphia became known as "the Great Triumvirate."
Working coöperatively, the heads of the three pioneer schools
wielded great power in the field of education of the blind.

5 OPENING OF NEW WAYS

HERE is no record that the early heads of either the New York or the Philadelphia schools ever became militant crusaders for the blind outside of their own bailiwicks. Certainly Russ and Friedlander were content to tread in the paths they created and were not, like Howe, "looking ever for something new." This may have been because the tenures of both were short and their schools therefore lacked the strength that came to Perkins through long unbroken leadership—three directors in one hundred years.

Certainly it was Howe who took the lead in urging the education of blind children in other parts of the country. Six months after he had opened the Boston school, he gave a public demonstration of his pupils before the Massachusetts General Court and thus began the practice of annual visits with his pupils to the legislatures of the New England States soliciting support. Considering his violent criticism of the Paris school for its "parades and shows," this must have meant some sacrifice of principle to the American pioneer. But by this time, Howe had but one concern, and that was to enlist interest in the blind and their potentialities wherever he could get a hearing.

In 1836, Howe set out on the first of a series of trips which, in the first decade of the Boston school, took him before the governing bodies of seventeen states. In that year, a letter from Dr. William M. Awl of Columbus, Ohio, asking for information about schooling for the blind, inspired Howe to set out with the two Carter girls and one other pupil to give a demonstration before the Ohio legislature. The exhibition proved so effective that "provision for the education of the blind was made before the representatives of the people had time to wipe the tears from their eyes."

Howe did more than move the legislators to tears. He sent to the Ohio school the necessary books, maps, and supplies and provided the first teacher, A. W. Penniman, the first graduate of the New England institution. Under Penniman's leadership, the little school opened on July 4, 1837, in the rooms of the First Presbyterian Church in Columbus. The significance of this event is that Ohio was the first state to make public provision for the education of its blind children.

In 1842, Dr. Howe set out with his troupe of actors for Kentucky, where they made a great impression on the legislators and citizens of that state. Immediately all who viewed the demonstration were in favor of opening a school. Communities vied with one another to be considered the most suitable site. Spontaneously, $10,000 was appropriated for the new work and so enthusiastic was Dr. Howe that he wrote Horace Mann: "The school in Louisville will probably be the largest in the country and will suffice for the southwestern states."

"I want to see these schools," he continued, "multiplied and magnified, not only for the blind alone, but for the influence they have upon the community by furnishing occasions for the exercise of the benevolent affections." [1] This is a letter that Dr. Howe may well have regretted writing, for he was wrong about both the size of the Louisville school and its sufficiency for the southwest, and later he spoke strongly against multiplying schools for the blind. But multiply they did under the impulse of the great humanitarian and through the exercise of the benevolent affections that were stirred up in many states.

By 1870, there were twenty-three schools and now there are fifty, making provision for the education of blind children in every state. All but six of these are state-supported and maintained institutions. Maryland in 1853, Pittsburgh in

1888, and Connecticut in 1893, joined the three pioneer schools as privately endowed and managed institutions, although all receive state aid in some form.

In eleven states, blind children and deaf children are educated in what are called "dual schools," a combination usually considered unfavorable to the blind pupils. The head of the dual school in Colorado, in protesting this plan in his report for 1908, stated the case effectively: "They [deaf and blind children] have nothing in common in the matter of education and the bringing of the two classes together is a prolific source of friction and compromise." Perhaps Ohio in the recent construction of two new schools has shown the extent to which efficient duality can be carried. Separate schools for the blind and for the deaf have been erected on adjoining properties with a central heating and service building serving both.

While residential schools have been for over a century the dominant form of education for blind children in this country, another form has been slowly emerging which at the present time is commanding increasing attention. This form is provided through day classes for blind children in the public schools. Started in this country a little more than half a century ago, day classes have been established chiefly in large cities. Until very recently, their enrollment has seldom exceeded 10 per cent of the total number of blind children in school, but in 1955 the ratio had advanced to 26 per cent.

As enrollments in the day classes have increased, the number of pupils in the residential schools has decreased from the peak enrollment of 6,032 in 1940. On January 3, 1955 there were 1,645 blind children attending day classes in 54 centers in 16 states. At the same time, there were enrolled in 52 residential schools, 5,794 blind pupils, plus 547 partially seeing children. The smaller number of schools than the 57 previously mentioned is due to the merger of several schools for the colored blind with those for white children.

The custom of educating sightless children in the common schools is almost as old as are the residential schools. Johann Klein, shortly after opening the school in Vienna in 1806, tried to have visually handicapped children admitted to the schools for the seeing, and from 1834 to 1836 blind pupils were placed in the classes for the seeing in Edinburgh. The first really successful effort to educate blind children in day classes was in Greenock, Scotland, in 1868. Soon thereafter, they were accommodated in the schools of Glasgow. In 1875, Dr. Alexander Barnhill of the Glasgow Mission to the Outdoor Blind was so enthusiastic about this type of education that he issued a pamphlet entitled *A New Era in the Education of Blind Children.*

In 1879, day classes for blind children were started by the London School Board and for sixteen years they had government support. In 1936, a survey was made and it was decided that there were not enough children to make the classes practical in any but urban areas. The report also stated: "We are of the opinion . . . that the education of blind children, especially young children, is of too specialized a character to permit of its being treated as an appendage to the scheme of education in the ordinary elementary schools." The law of 1944 requires all blind children in England to be educated in residential schools, and in Scotland the education act of 1950 recommends that all blind children attend the Royal Blind School in Edinburgh. There are still day classes for the blind in Germany. The first class was started in 1878 in Berlin and placed in a building adjoining a school for training domestics so that the girls could escort the blind children to and from school.

The first day class in this country was opened in Chicago on September 17, 1900. It came about through the demand of parents for educational facilities for their blind children nearer to home than the state school at Jacksonville, which is in the southern part of the state. Land had been acquired and plans ordered for building a second residential school when Frank H. Hall, superintendent of the Illinois State School for the Blind; Edward J. Nolan, a blind lawyer who was a graduate of the state school; and John B. Curtis, who had attended the Illinois School but was graduated from a public high school in Chicago and from the University of

Chicago, approached the Board of Education and persuaded them to open as an experiment a day class for blind children in a school for the seeing. Mr. Curtis became the first teacher and continued in the work until 1935.

During the half century, most classes in public schools followed the pattern established in Chicago, where a room was set apart under a special teacher but insofar as possible the blind pupils shared in the classes of the seeing. Cincinnati opened a class in 1905 where the blind were segregated from the seeing, but in 1913 it adopted the coöperative plan. In Cleveland, where braille classes were introduced in 1909, Robert B. Irwin, the first supervisor, did much to supplement the regular program by asking the blind pupils to come to school on Saturday mornings for extra instruction in music and crafts, the lack of which was a shortcoming of the early day classes. The teachers supervised the pupils' table manners at lunch, took them on week-end hikes, and organized a summer camp, to which the parents were also invited for instruction.

New York City opened braille classes in 1909 as a part of Superintendent W. H. Maxwell's plan to make provision in the program of public education for all handicapped children. Detroit opened its first day class in 1912 and for a time rented a house near the school for girls who lived too far away to come daily. Los Angeles, when in 1917 it made provision for the education of the visually handicapped in its public-school system, placed them in a separate school, thereby depriving the children of close association in the classroom with seeing boys and girls. In 1919, classes were begun in Minneapolis and St. Paul, and in the following year Seattle opened a class. This was at first coöperative but later, when it changed to the segregated type, most of the pupils returned to the residential school.

New Jersey, which has never maintained a residential school, was the first to provide state support and supervision of braille classes, making them the accepted method of education for their blind children. This plan was initiated by Lydia Y. Hayes, the first supervisor of the blind in that state and a Perkins graduate. It must be added, however, that New Jersey calls frequently on the residential schools of neighboring states and that at least one-third of her visually handicapped children normally are in residence in them. "Our blind children," wrote George F. Meyer, the present head of the work for the blind in New Jersey, "from the beginning develop the concept that they are, primarily, citizens of the school or of the community, and only secondarily, blind." [2]

This review of the beginnings and the development of educational facilities for blind childern in this country reveals that at the persent time there are available three forms of education, as pointed out in a recent publication of the American Foundation for the Blind:

1. Education in a public, parochial, or private residential school for the blind;

2. Education with the sighted in a public, parochial, or private school, with a resource teacher or a braille class teacher available during the entire school day;

3. Education with sighted children in a public, parochial, or private school with itinerant supervision by a resource teacher available at regular or needed intervals.

The statement continues that "not for a long time, if ever, will any one of these three patterns suffice to the exclusion of the others."

Little has been said of the third pattern, but it refers to the fact that a number of parents are entering their blind children in nursery schools for seeing children and sometimes continuing them in seeing schools through their whole educational career. A more common form is the growing practice of some residential schools, when circumstances warrant it, of sending children back to their homes to attend the local school under the supervision of itinerant teachers. These are specialists in the education of the blind who travel from school to school in a community system.

Other residential schools encourage advanced and well-qualified students to attend a nearby high school for class work while providing suitable texts and supervision of study.

This plan has become so well accepted that a number of schools for the blind no longer maintain high-school departments. The practice began in 1890, when Newell Perry, a student attending the California School for the Blind, asked to be permitted to attend the adjacent high school for his academic work. After graduation from the high school, he went on to the University of California, did graduate work in Germany and at Columbia University, and then returned to the California School, where for many years he was its able principal.

Perusal of the reports of the American Association of Instructors of the Blind in earlier years indicates that, at first, heads of the residential schools feared that the day classes might lead to their liquidation, and more recently the social workers are blamed for this deviation from the traditional pattern of education for blind youth. It is therefore of interest to note that among the first to deplore weaknesses in the congregate plan and to see promise in the day classes were enlightened leaders of residential schools whose primary concern was the welfare of blind children. They became concerned when they realized that too many of their pupils, after years of separation from their families and home communities, were finding it difficult to take the contributory place in life that was the main objective of their education.

Reading through Dr. Howe's reports, which became guide books for educators of the blind, it is of value to note a change in his attitude toward the residential school which the proponents of that system have not always been ready to recognize. In 1850, he wrote:

I am most ready to acknowledge that my views respecting the organization of establishments, even for the education of ordinary youth, have materially changed. I think that all the advantages arising from them may be gained, and most of the crying evils attendant upon them avoided, by breaking up the "common system," boarding the youth among families in the neighborhood, and bringing them together daily for purposes of instruction and for the advantages of mutual action of their minds upon each other . . . This system would be more costly, in a pecuniary point of view, than the present one; so much more that it will hardly be adopted in our generation.[3]

In 1851, Dr. Howe wrote at length of the dangers

when a hundred of these [blind] children are brought together in an institution formed for training and instructing them in common . . . A clannish spirit begins to appear, and to increase, the longer the association continues. We see the seeds of the evil in our institutions; and we see the full fruit, in all its deformity, in the great asylums of Europe which the blind inhabit for life . . . Our own establishment having been the first organized in this country, we, at least, had no profit of the experience of any but European institutions, and upon these we certainly have made some improvements, of which they have since availed themselves. There is room for still more improvement . . . But in administering our institutions, we are met at the outset by a difficulty which makes me fear there is a fundamental error in their organization. During the six or seven years in which the character is most easily moulded, the blind must associate almost exclusively with each other, whereas we have seen that it is most desirable that they should associate with the seeing.[4]

On September 6, 1866, Samuel Gridley Howe made the address at the laying of the cornerstone of the New York Institution for the Blind in Batavia. The officials who invited him, and indeed the officers of many of the other residential schools who were undoubtedly there, must have regretted this choice when Howe said: "I would observe, by the way, that the necessity now felt for a new institution in your state has arisen, partly at least, from radical faults in the organization of the old one, such as I have noticed." He then cited the evils that he had observed, pointed out the things that should have been done, and stated: "If these things had been done, the State would perhaps not now be called upon to incur the cost and the continual expense of carrying on a second institution."

In this address, Howe made a statement that all who are opposed to residential schools like to quote:

All great establishments in the nature of boarding schools, where the sexes must be separated; where there must be boarding in common, and sleeping in congregate dormitories; where there must be routine, and formality, and restraint, and repression of individuality; where the charms and refining influences of the true family relation cannot be had,—all such institutions are unnatural, undesirable, and very liable to abuse. We should have as few of them as is possible, and those few should be kept as small as possible.

The human family is the unit of society. The family, as it was ordained by our Great Father, with its ties of kith and kin; with its tender associations of childhood and youth; with its ties of affection and of sympathy; with its fireside, its table, and its domestic altar,—there is the place for the early education of the child. His instruction may be had in school; his heart and character should be developed and moulded at home.[5]

Dr. Howe's concern for blind children taken from their homes and the normal ties of kith and kin was very genuine, and, shortly after his return from administering relief in Crete in 1868, he took steps to alleviate the deplored circumstances of congregate living. In this, he was spurred to action by Dr. Edward Jarvis, a former associate of Howe in Greece and at the time a trustee of Perkins; in fact, he was in charge of the Institution while the Director was in Crete.

In Dr. Jarvis's report to the trustees for 1868, he wrote:

The sole object of this Institution is to take these persons of impaired or extinct vision and so to teach, educate, and train them that, as far as possible, they shall know the facts and apprehend the principles that are taught to others, and that they shall have power to give and receive employment in society, to engage in the work and business of the great world abroad, and sustain themselves in health and strength, and discharge responsibilities of individual and social life . . .

The apparent necessity and the actual custom of separating the blind children and youth from their homes and families . . . and gathering them into exclusive families and schools of their own sort in institutions deprives them of these opportunities of public education in common schools with the numbers and varieties of others, in the street with the miscellaneous children of the neighborhood and town, at home and in friends' homes with persons of all ages, pursuits, and purposes.[6]

Under the impulse of the Jarvis report, plans for the re-building of Perkins were evidently taken under serious consideration, for Dr. Howe in his report for the following year outlined plans that called for the elimination of the congregate system of living and the erection of separate cottages for small groups of pupils. Through this system, Howe hoped to obtain more effective separation of the sexes and to secure greater facilities for classifying the pupils both in school and in the houses. Dr. Jarvis commended the new plan as "a decided step in the advance toward completeness in the education of the blind, and in their preparation to meet the responsibilities of life."

"Perhaps," he added, "it is as great a step as we, in the present generation, are prepared to take." But he expressed the hope that in another generation

another step will be taken in this direction, and all the blind children of the city will be left in their several homes. Then but not until then, these sightless children will have opportunities for complete development and education as nearly equal to those enjoyed by their more favored brothers and sisters, as their peculiar disability will allow.[7]

Financial difficulties made it impossible to carry out the full plan or reorganization worked out by Howe and Jarvis, but in 1870 the trustees of Perkins built two double houses which were occupied by the girls as four family groups. The boys and a few men employed in the workshop continued to live in the dormitories of the old hotel. By this action, Dr. Howe is generally credited with originating the noncongregate or cottage plan of institutional living now considered standard in the best social institutions. But both he and Dr. Jarvis looked upon this as a first step toward the ideal.

Michael Anagnos, a young Greek who had assisted Dr. Howe in Crete, came back with him, became a teacher at Perkins, and married his daughter. In 1876, he succeeded Howe as the second director of the Boston school. Although practically in full charge of the Institution during the last years of the first director, he did not fully share Dr. Howe's

concern for the dangers of congregate living, and the multiplying of such institutions.

Indeed, he added another when in 1887 he founded the
Kindergarten, the first of its kind in the world. This took
little blind children out of their homes at the age of five
and during their most impressionable years added four years
to the program of congregate living and schooling. Anagnos,
however, did heed his father-in-law's injunction about living
in large groups, for he built the new school at Jamaica Plain
around small house units. But perhaps his most significant
contribution was that he removed the pecuniary obstacle that
made Howe feel that his ideal plan could not be carried out
in his generation. For Anagnos had a phenomenal gift of
luring money out of benevolent citizens of Massachusetts.
So persuasive was he that proper Bostonians of his day would
hardly dare face Saint Peter unless they had made provision
for Perkins in their wills, a fact that greatly eased the financial problems of his successors.

Attending the 1886 convention of the American Association of Instructors of the Blind, Anagnos revealed his faith
in the residential school when he said:

These institutions are founded upon the solid rock of equity,
and not upon the piers of pity or of charity. They derive the means
of their support from unfailing sources, and constitute important
links in the magnificent chain of public education, which encircles
and binds together and solidifies this great republic. They have
aimed at the attainment of practical results, and have aided the
recipients of their advantages to rise above the clouds of ignorance
and superstition and to breathe the air of independence on the
heights of activity and social equality.[8]

Michael Anagnos' successor, Edward Ellis Allen, who took
office in 1906 and who rounded out a century of leadership
at Perkins under three directors, was more concerned than
his predecessor about the dangers of congregate living, and
at the outset he determined to remove them. Immediately he
resolved to take the Institution out of the "abandoned hotel
turned over to the blind" and with the money raised by
Anagnos to reconstruct Perkins on a garden site. He had al-

ready done this at Philadelphia, but as he often said, "I profited by the mistakes that I made there."

The new plant, completed in Watertown in 1913, consists of two separate sections. Eight cottages planned to house the older students from the Institution in South Boston are grouped around a central school building bearing the name of the first director. This is now known as the Upper School. Four combined living and school units with auditorium, library, and gymnasium for the Kindergarten from Jamaica Plain (now known as the Lower School) surround a quadrangle named after the second director. The cottages were designed to simulate family life, with a matron in charge of each and a master in residence in houses for boys. Most of the sleeping rooms are for two pupils, with some single rooms and a few for three occupants. Teachers live in the cottages and eat their meals with the pupils in the cottage dining room. In this way, Dr. Allen carried to full fruition the cottage plan begun by Dr. Howe in 1870. But he retained the residential-school principle.

6 THE WAY AHEAD

HE significance of the new Perkins plant at Watertown is that it set the standard which for nearly half a century has dominated the schools for the blind in the United States and to a limited degree those in other countries. As new schools were erected or enlarged, they tried to emulate, insofar as finances would permit, the cottage plan of Perkins. New York, however, when it built its new buildings on Pelham Parkway, continued dormitory living and retained a central dining room, as Dr. Allen had done in his rebuilding of the Philadelphia school.

Maryland, in moving to Overlea, built around Newcomb Hall, the central school building, small separate cottages for its pupils, much smaller than the living units at Perkins. John F. Bledsoe, the superintendent, was fond of chiding Dr. Allen about referring to his rows of manor houses as cottages. Other schools, notably Ohio in its rebuilding and the New York School at Batavia, in its expansion, have gone a long way from the old deplored system of congregate living. And yet one cannot but wonder what that pattern might have been if Dr. Allen had taken up the full challenge of Howe and Jarvis to the next generation, to place blind children in the common schools, and had thrown the prestige of Perkins behind it.

In his rebuilding and in his conduct of the new Perkins, Dr. Allen continued wholeheartedly Dr. Howe's policy of the segregation of the sexes. Not only were the pupils housed in cottages for boys and cottages for girls, but in the school buildings the males and the females were separated by an invisible but impenetrable wall; this wall has since been gradually whittled down by his successors. Dr. Allen, however, heeding the counsel of Dr. Jarvis, did a great deal to provide opportunity for the blind pupils to have social contacts with seeing boys and girls both within and outside of the school.

In his later years, Dr. Allen made statements which many felt to be an acknowledgment that perhaps the residential schools lacked something that the public school classes had to offer blind youth preparing to take places as contributors in the seeing world. For he wrote in 1938, seven years after his retirement:

> Certainly I would place a blind child of five or six years in a public or private kindergarten, if I could. This is no experiment; it has been done and with surprising benefit also to the seeing tots. Yes, and I could cite instances where wisely guided blind pupils got all their schooling among the seeing, and never regretted it.

And also:

> But,—this very possibility of continuously motivated entertainment within a cloistered, self-serving, self-sufficient community has its weak if not its bad side. Because it does not furnish the pupils with enough brushes with reality . . . because it fits but poorly for quick diffusion in the world outside . . . If I could plan and carry out my preference now, I should conduct no senior high school department but would send every proper pupil of that advancement out daily for such opportunities or, if conditions favored, bring about such individual's attendance at the high school of his own town.[1]

These concessions, expressed by one who for a quarter of a century was the head of one of the pioneer schools for the blind in this country, are illustrative of a change of attitude that is growing among educators of the blind and is more aggressively expressed by social workers. George F. Meyer, executive officer of the New Jersey State Commission for the Blind and a leading exponent of day classes, states:

> These changes merely reflect an adaptation on the part of residential schools to a change in attitude of thinking people toward

institutional care for children, a more universal appreciation of social factors in education, and a general broadening of educational philosophy.

The general conception that institutional care should be substituted for life in the family and the community only as a last resort, has been gaining ground in the social treatment of persons of all ages.[2]

From the social point of view, nearly everyone will grant that the right place for any child is in the home, and, as Mr. Meyer stated, institutionalism should be only a last resort. And yet the prevailing pattern for the schooling of nine-tenths of the blind children in this country, and in other parts of the world almost entirely, has been to take them from their families and place them in residential schools.

Nearly one hundred years ago, Dr. Howe decried this practice, asserting that if separation from the home is necessary there should be small, intimate units simulating family life for all children handicapped physically, mentally, or emotionally. Perhaps Dr. Thomas D. Cutsforth, author of *The Blind in School and Society,* had a point when he said: "There was enough of the sage and of the scientist in that grand old abolitionist [Howe] that if he should make a centennial visit to America, he would be the first to apply the torch to much of his own construction." [3]

From the educational viewpoint, the story is different. It is probably true that most, if not all, of the residential schools for the blind have educational standards at least as high as the common schools of their respective states. Some are far superior in equipment, in the quality of instruction, and in the caliber of their teachers. This, of course, is usually true of boarding schools for the seeing. That is why many educators of the blind are honest in their reluctance to give way to the day classes. They want their pupils to have the best and it is true that many blind boys and girls receive a far better education in the residential schools than do their seeing brothers and sisters in the public schools of their communities.

This also raises a serious question which the residential schools must meet. Is it right to give handicapped youth education that they will not have the opportunity to use? Today too many visually handicapped young people seek higher education rather than face work at a level at which they have a better chance to compete. Too many, after years of adulation for their achievements in the university, conclude their working careers by the frustration of the sheltered shop. That was what bothered Samuel Gridley Howe. Education of the blind in his time was outrunning the opportunities for employment made available by the seeing. For his early graduates, Howe had to build a shop. He was, therefore, interested in a new educational scheme which gave promise of keeping the blind integrated with the seeing during their growing years and thereby opening larger possibilities to find employment and to become contributors.

The fact that most of the residential schools have better facilities for education confronts the advocates of the day classes with a situation that they must face realistically. For it may be said without equivocation that the residential schools will not advise parents to send their children to day classes until there is strong evidence that the public schools are able to provide programs with adequate facilities, competent teachers, and the spirit to give that extra lift which handicapped children need.

This calls not only for an understanding administration of matters pertaining to the curriculum but also for assurance of a full integration of blind pupils into all phases of school life. Isolation in an environment of noncoöperating pupils and unsympathetic teachers can be more frustrating to blind children than education away from home in a school where house mothers and teachers understand their special problems and where they will be among their peers.

Steps to come to a better understanding of the problems involved in the education of the handicapped child, or, as the experts say, the exceptional child, are being taken in several areas. Nearly all state departments of education and many universities now have divisions of special education concerned with the well-being of atypical children. And in the field of the blind, studies of problems of special education from the visual angle are being undertaken. Such a project was the National Work Session on the Education of the Blind with the Sighted, held August 24–28, 1953, at Pine Brook Camp, Upper Saranac Lake, New York. Sponsored by the American Foundation for the Blind and with the coöperation of the Department for the Education of Exceptional Children, Syracuse University, at whose camp the conference was held, a group of workers in this field discussed problems that they have encountered in their work.

The report of the gathering presents constructively a wealth of background and material in this field and a compilation of resources and equipment that will have value. Leaders of the residential schools may well feel that the discussions at the work session might have been more realistic if they have been invited, for they could have pointed out to the group some of the problems they have encountered in the boys and girls who have come to them after failure in the public schools due largely to the present inadequacy in many places. Dr. William M. Cruikshank, head of the Department for Education of Exceptional Children at Syracuse, stated well the attitude needed in these discussions when he said:

The question of the residential school and/or the public day school class is undecided in the minds of many professional people . . . these are issues which intellectually mature people should approach with logic and with the confidence that solutions can be reached. It is up to us in education for exceptional children to put our own house in order immediately.[4]

The good advice of this distinguished teacher can well be taken in the field of the blind. While the residential schools have a record of achievement of which they can be justly proud, there are certain suggestions that can be made to their leaders if they are to hold their place in serving blind youth. For example, if schooling among their peers is one of the strong claims of the residential schools, their proponents must be on their guard against weakening that position by the growing tendency to lower visual requirements so that partially seeing boys and girls may be admitted. This has gone so far that two schools have eliminated the world "blind" from their names. It is not a new problem, for in 1866, at the dedication of the school at Batavia, New York, Dr. Howe warned against it, pointing out that from 10 to 15 percent of the pupils in schools for the blind had too much sight to be there.

The survey made by the first White House Conference on Child Health and Welfare in 1931 revealed that "in forty-four schools, having a total enrollment of 4,195, there were 673 students (16 percent) having sufficient vision to permit their reading inkprint." In 1950, federal government authorities responsible for the funds provided to the American Printing House for the Blind for braille books and appliances for schools ruled that allocation of the money must be on the basis of legally blind pupils and not on total enrollments. In that year, enrollments totalled 5,757 of whom 743 were not legally blind, and by the ruling of the federal government were not entitled to share in the funds designated to help in the education of blind children.

The presence in residential schools of these partially seeing pupils may be attributed to the best of motives: to the poor visual prognosis of an entering pupil, to recognition of the lack of sight-saving class facilities in rural areas, to the need of the all-round program of the residential school, and sometimes to the fact that after a pupil has entered the school his eye condition has improved. In these days when applications for admission to schools for the blind are increasing owing to the number of children becoming blind through premature birth, it might be wise to look into this way of making room for their accommodation. But the present tendency to accept partially seeing children in residential schools for the blind is a questionable practice from the point of view of modern education, even if they are provided with sight-saving books, and equipment from other sources.

This matter was carefully considered by a competent committee of the National Society for the Prevention of Blindness (within whose area of interest all work for the partially seeing has historically rested) which after outlining four methods of placement—(1) in schools for the blind, (2) in special schools providing for all handicapped groups, (3) in segregated classes in public schools, and (4) in coöperative classes—endorsed the fourth.[5] That method differs from the third in that the partially seeing pupils join seeing classmates in all activities not requiring continued use of eyes. For concentrated eye work, there is a well-equipped classroom with a specially trained teacher in charge. In all placements, there must always be considerable flexibility, especially in cases of children with borderline vision.

Leaders of the residential schools are opening themselves to the suspicion of trying to counterbalance the drop in enrollment not only by raising the visual acuity limit but also by lowering the age for admission. The recent tendency to make provision for blind children commonly described as of preschool age seems to be spreading. To admit such children to residential schools is to run counter to the experience of the past in the field of education of the blind and to the modern concept of child welfare. All thoughtful people accept the principle that the proper place for the young child is in the home, and experience has shown that the warmth of family care even in a poor home is often better than the best institutional care.

In England, where the long-established provision for the care of the infant blind has been the nursery home, there has been a change in attitude, for the 1952 report of the Royal National Institute for the Blind states: "A good home is always the best place for a very young child, but housing or other domestic problems sometimes makes the upbringing of a blind child difficult. In such a case, the child can be sent to one of the Royal National Institute's Sunshine Home Nursery Schools."

The first nursery for blind babies (not by any means a nursery school in the modern sense) was opened in Hartford in 1893. Others soon followed, but all have closed their doors except the Boston Nursery for Blind Babies, which has amplified its program to provide a varied service for babies and their mothers. In 1950, a nursery school was opened in Los Angeles. Although it provides for a few boarders, it is primarily a day school. The accepted practice in this country is to help the parents of blind babies provide for their care in their own homes. Many state commissions for the blind now include on their staffs visiting teachers who go into the homes to advise in the care of blind babies, and to suggest or provide needed equipment.

Many schools for the blind now hold summer institutes to which parents and babies are invited for instruction and for what is often a by-product of greater importance—the exchange of experiences among mothers coping with a common problem. This is a good and rightful contribution for schools for the blind to make for this age group. Certainly it is better than retrogression to a discarded practice which, while relieving some mothers of their problems, does so at the cost of the child's right to the security of home and the warmth of parental affection.

Another aspect of change that is decidedly encouraging and has potential value is the interest now found among the parents of visually handicapped children and in the homes from which they come, either to enter the residential schools or to attend the day classes. In former days, it was often said that blind children came from substandard homes and that their parents were unable or unwilling to cope with them. There was a large measure of truth in that attitude, but it has far less validity today. Homes are now better, or can be made better through competent social work, and the attitudes of parents have changed from apathy to aggressive concern for their handicapped children.

One of the most powerful and promising forces in the field of the blind today is the spontaneous growth of organized groups of parents of blind children. Perhaps the future plans for the education of blind youth will depend not on the discussions or deliberations of educators in either camp, but rather on the determination of parents whose children are the factors of ultimate concern. As a consequence of all these forces, residential schools for the blind are beginning to reappraise their programs in accordance with present needs and in order to be able to offer wider opportunities for the education of blind children from which parents may make a choice.

In 1941, the Oregon School for the Blind announced a new plan whereby that residential school, in coöperation with the Department of Education, would serve as a clearinghouse for all cases of visually handicapped children in the state. On recommendation of the Division of Special Education, children would be accepted at the school in Salem, their problems and needs diagnosed, and a plan of education best adapted to their needs developed. Some would remain at the school, others would be sent to either the braille or sight-saving classes within the state, while still others might be returned to their regular schools with special instructions for their schooling.

Five years after the inauguration of this plan, Superintendent Walter R. Dry reported:

It is not only possible, but entirely feasible to correlate the work of the residential school and the public school. Such a program is not inimical to the interest of the children without sight or those with low vision. Rather, it will give these children much-needed experience in living in a world to which they must eventually adjust. Furthermore, it should serve to give the public school children—our citizens of tomorrow—a better understanding of the problem and the potentialities of those who are without sight.[6]

The most recent and perhaps the most comprehensive plan to provide blind children with "the widest choice of a program" is that proposed in September 1953, by the present director of Perkins Institution, Edward J. Waterhouse, under the name of "The New England Plan." This calls for the formation of a five-state "New England Council for the Education of the Blind" with representatives from Perkins Institution and the appropriate state departments of education or public welfare. "It is our philosophy," wrote Mr. Waterhouse,

that the educational program should be fitted to the child, and not the child to the program.

For many (and possibly for all blind children at some age in their school careers), the residential school is the best solution. In addition to the special courses and trained personnel, there are opportunities for widespread competition on an equal footing, and an escape during difficult periods of growth from being a conspicuously unique member of the group. For many, the security of the home, family, and neighbors is more important, and these should have opportunity to be educated in the public schools.[7]

Under this plan, blind children, after careful consideration of many factors pertaining to their welfare, will be assigned to the most suitable form of education. Perkins proposed to train teachers, provide equipment, give training in areas not covered in the day classes, and make available such supervision of the public-school work as the authorities may request. All of which seems a way to strengthen the weak spots in many day-class programs. And this is from Perkins, a pioneer residential school. Dr. Howe would be pleased!

Howe's report of Perkins Institution for 1874 is considered his valedictory, for in it he reviewed the past and expressed his hopes for the future. "It has been shown in many cases," he wrote, "that blind children can attend common schools advantageously, and be instructed in classes with normal children. They labor under certain disadvantages" which he proceeded to point out, but "on the other hand, they have certain advantages, and become fashioned and fitted for future social relations, as they cannot be in a school filled with blind children." Howe told of observing mute children being taught in the district schools of France and stated that he attempted to introduce the same methods here,

but unfortunately pressure of business prevented my devoting to the matter the time and attention necessary to success.

I made a beginning, however, and . . . I trust that others, with more zeal and vigor than I have left, will put this into practice, until it shall be the custom to send to the common school such blind children as do not need the special attention and instruction which can only be had in institutions calculated to meet their wants. The practice of training and teaching a considerable proportion of blind and mute children in the common schools is to be one of the improvements of the future.[8]

To understand Howe's hope that blind and mute children could be educated in the schools of their home communities, one must not forget that Horace Mann, the ardent proponent of the common education of all children in publicly supported schools, was his closest friend. Together they took their brides to Europe on their honeymoons and together they waged battle against the social and educational ills of their time. Mann believed and advocated that every child has a right to free education, provided by the community without any semblance of segregation because of wealth, color, religion, or physical infirmity.

As this movement grew, the pioneer educator of the blind in America gave his support and, because of the indomitable conviction of his friend Horace Mann, Samuel Gridley Howe came to feel not only that the principle was right but that here was a way to avoid the evils of congregate living which he decried and the segregation of blind children from their families which he deplored. Instruction of all children, including the handicapped, in the common schools would provide opportunity for those with visual impairment to grow up in the warmth of family life, in the security of the home community, and thereby, through their natural association with those who knew them, the gate would be opened more widely for employment and contribution.

This was the hope that Howe proclaimed in his last years. "It will hardly come in my day," he wrote two years before he died, "but I see it plainly with the eye of faith; and rejoice in the prospect of its fulfillment." Schools have changed since that time. Contrast the little schoolhouse of a century ago and its lack of facilities for special education, with the present consolidated school, with specialists in all areas, shops, bands, home economics, free lunches, and medical care.

Nearly nine million public-school children, one out of three, now ride to their classes in school busses and a million more use private automobiles, thereby eliminating the old hazard of travel. Homes are better equipped to deal with handicapped children, and parents dominate the schools through strong organizations. And the rising costs of operating the residential schools, coupled with the possibilities of decreasing enrollments, reverse the situation of 1850, when the old pioneer feared that the new way "would be more costly, in a pecuniary point of view, than the present one; so much more that it will hardly be adopted in our generation." Perhaps the time has come, in America, at least, for the fulfillment or certainly for a fuller consideration of the high hopes of Samuel Gridley Howe—the Cadmus of the blind.

7 CHILDREN OF THE SILENT NIGHT

U P to this point, consideration has been given only to children with impaired vision. Among these, however, are many who have other deviations which call for even more specialized forms of instruction. For some blind children are, and in about the same ratio as seeing children, also retarded mentally or handicapped physically. And in many of these cases it is difficult to determine which is the major barrier to adequate instruction. Should the crippled blind child go to the school for crippled children or to the school for the blind? Are the physical aspects of the cardiac or the diabetic more demanding of attention than his intellectual needs? These are problems with which modern special education is wrestling and the answers have not yet been determined.

Even in the one field of special education where achievement has been spectacular—the deaf-blind—there is ambivalence as to whether the major defect is the loss of hearing or the loss of sight. Historically and technically, schools for the deaf, especially those using the oral method, are better equipped from the point of view of instruction than schools for the blind to reach the imprisoned minds of those who are both deaf and blind. But from the earliest times educators of the deaf, while often speculating about the possibility, have hesitated to come to grips with the problem and until very recently have taken an "out-of-bounds" attitude.

Thus it has happened that in this country, at least, most of the outstanding work with deaf-blind children has been achieved by educators of the blind. This may be attributed to the indomitable spirit of Samuel Gridley Howe, whose success with Laura Bridgman has been hailed as one of the wonders of the educational world. Laura, triply handicapped, came to Perkins in 1837 and under Howe's tutelage became the first deaf-blind mute to acquire the use of language. Since that time, there has been an unceasing stream of doubly and often triply handicapped children at the Massachusetts school, where they are now known as The Children of the Silent Night.

While Samuel Gridley Howe is historically credited with being the first to adapt successfully methods of education to the needs of the deaf-blind, there is an interesting story of earlier concern and speculation. Its pattern follows closely the first interest in the possibility of educating the sightless, but it does not come to the same constructive conclusion. There was no Jean Jacques Rousseau to throw down a challenge of action to the speculators. In England in 1648 a book was published which states "that a man borne Blinde, Deafe and Dumbe, may be taught to heare the sound of words with his eies and thence to learne to speake with his tongue . . . For the truth is, they speak not, because they cannot hear." It also relates, without explanation, "that one Anagildus, who was reported both deafe and dumbe and blinde was restored to all his senses, whilst he prayed unto St. Julian." [1] The indicated author of this book, "J. B. surnamed the Chrisapher," was probably Dr. John Bulwer, the first Englishman to be interested in the deaf.

More than a century later, the Abbé Deschamps, a Frenchman, in a book published in 1779, outlined a method of instructing deaf-blind children by first teaching them speech through the proper placement of lips and tongue. In 1795, a woman in England is said to have learned to communicate "by talking with her fingers, at which she was uncommonly ready," and in the same year a book was printed in Madrid setting forth a method of teaching the deaf-blind through the senses of touch, smell, and taste.

"I would compose," the author, Lorenzo Heuvas y Pandura, wrote,

> a spelling book of letters in high relief; I should have the blind-deaf mute touch them with his fingers. Then I would present to him the word "bread" in raised letters; I would have him take a piece of bread and taste it and in this way I would make him understand what the word "bread" meant . . . And so the mind of the deaf-blind would acquire knowledge . . . for experience shows that the knowledge of the deaf-blind is as if dammed up. It is manifested at first very slowly, but as soon as it is aroused, it runs rapidly like a torrent which has been held in restraint.[2]

The Spanish writer indicated that the Abbé de L'Epée (founder of the work for the deaf in France) tried to find a blind deaf-mute to see if he could teach him. If he had succeeded in doing so, the Spanish author stated, "he would have acquired no small glory." It is true that de L'Epée did have an interest in the doubly handicapped, stimulated, no doubt, by Diderot's assertion, that the deaf-blind could be taught through touch by patient and persistent connection of tangible signs and objects. Although the founder of work for the deaf in France made no recorded progress with the deaf-blind, he did speculate on a method of teaching.

It remained for de L'Epée's successor, the Abbé Sicard, to expound a complete system for the instruction of those deprived of sight and hearing which followed in principle the method proposed by the Spanish author in 1795. This, however, was motivated primarily by a fear that some of his deaf mutes might lose their sight, the essential sense for lip reading. Sicard had no concern for deaf-blind children and after perfecting his system there was no clarion call for its application, for he wrote: "May such a system of education be only an object of rare speculation and its application never become necessary! May no child ever be born so unfortunate as to have instead of the ear and the eye, only the hand!" [3]

Another similarity to the pattern which led to the education of the blind is found in a deaf-blind boy in Scotland in 1795. In a way, James Mitchell may be considered the counterpart of the blind boy in England whose sight was restored through an operation. This resolved the speculations of the French philosophers and, it will be recalled, culminated in action and achievement. But the intense interest aroused through the widely heralded accounts of the deaf-blind boy in Scotland led only to negative conclusions. Although those who made a study of his case admitted that "Mitchell's mind displays a great share of native strength and is destitute only of the vehicles of its exhibition, the eyes and the ears," Sir Dugald Stuart and Sir Astley Cooper reported in 1812 to the Royal Society of Edinburgh that their work with James Mitchell indicated that the deaf-blind were uneducable.

The British report undoubtedly reached Dr. Howe in America. He must have heard of the speculations of the French abbés while in Paris, and the Spanish book with Howe's signature on the flyleaf is in the Perkins Library. To the intrepid American always looking for new fields to conquer, these were challenges that could not be ignored. And so when the pioneer educator of the blind heard of a deaf-blind girl, Julia Brace, at the American Asylum for the Deaf at Hartford, he lost no time in going to see her. The educators of the deaf had not succeeded in penetrating the barriers that imprisoned her mind, but Dr. Howe concluded "that the trial should not be abandoned, although it had failed in her case as well as in all that had been recorded before."

It is not difficult to imagine the eagerness of Dr. Howe when shortly after his visit to Julia Brace he learned of a child reported to be deaf, blind, and mute living in Etna, New Hampshire, seven miles outside of Hanover, the seat of Dartmouth College. The discovery of the triply handicapped child came through a student, James Barrett, who had been engaged by the selectmen of the town to make out tax bills during the month of May. While engaged in this work in the farmhouse of Daniel Bridgman, Barrett saw the child Laura with sightless eyes and speechless lips. Returning to college, he told Dr. Reuben Dimond Mussey, Secretary-Treasurer of the Medical School, about her, and he wrote an account for the press. This came to Dr. Howe's attention. His interest was immediately aroused and he lost little time in making the journey to the New Hampshire town.

The parents were soon persuaded by Dr. Howe that he could help their daughter. The only person who objected was Asa Tenney, an eccentric old bachelor, who was Laura's first friend and playmate. When no one else would have much to do with the severely handicapped child, Uncle Asa, as he was called, was always ready to take her on walks. Leading her to the brook near the house and making her put her hand in the running stream, he soon taught Laura the difference between earth and water. By a system of their own, Laura gained a knowledge of trees and flowers. After the talk with Dr. Howe, the parents soon realized that there was need for more definite work with their child. So on October 4, 1837, Mr. and Mrs. Bridgman and Laura left Hanover for Boston, where the deaf-blind child was enrolled at the New England Asylum for the Blind.

Since no method of instructing a child devoid of sight and hearing, the chief mediums of learning, had brought successful results, Dr. Howe was faced with the momentous problem of deciding how to begin and what medium to employ.

There was one of two ways to be adopted [wrote Dr. Howe]: either to go on and build up a language of signs on the basis of the natural language which she had already herself commenced; or to teach her the purely arbitrary language in common use: that is, to give her a sign for every individual thing, or to give her a knowledge of letters, by the combination of which she might express her idea of the existence, and the mode and condition of existence, of anything. The former would have been easy, but very ineffectual; the latter seemed very difficult, but if accomplished, very effectual. I determined, therefore, to try the latter.[4]

This theory was sound and simple. But how convey the idea of letters and the combination of letters to a deaf, blind child? Here Dr. Howe may have been helped by the method proposed by the Spanish educator. Howe had already devised an embossed line type for the blind to read with their fingers, and taking common objects of daily use, a key and a spoon, and later a knife and a book, he attached to these objects labels bearing their names in raised letters. The child was made to feel these objects and the words designating them until she associated name with object. The next step was to detach the labels from the objects, and the pupil, given an object, was taught to find the right name for it.

The third step was to place embossed letters before the child and have her select those that formed the name of the object given to her. A long, slow, tedious process, but it worked; and, pressing on step by step, Laura Bridgman learned to use words like a normal person, and to employ language to express thoughts and ideas. From a hopeless handicapped child she grew to be one of the most widely known women in the world. Laura learned to write with a pencil, and her daily journal is one of the chief measures of her progress, but she never learned to talk, even though Dr. Howe believed it would have been possible if he had had time to teach her.

Many visitors came to Perkins from all parts of the world to see this phenomenal girl, but perhaps the most notable was Charles Dickens, who visited the school with Charles Sumner in Januray 1842. So interested was Dickens, that, as a teacher recorded, he "did not deign to notice anything or anybody except Laura." In his *American Notes,* Dickens devoted fourteen of the thirty pages given to Boston to a description of Perkins Institution and the education of Laura Bridgman.

Some forty years later, the reading of this account of the education of Laura Bridgman in the *American Notes,* by a woman in Alabama formed the first link of a chain that reaches into the present day. New hope flooded the heart of the reader, for she had a child also deprived of sight and hearing. This was Helen Keller, then six years old. Contact was soon made through Alexander Graham Bell with Michael Anagnos, the second director of Perkins Institution, and it was arranged that a teacher, trained in the methods successfully used with Laura Bridgman, should be sent to the Alabama home. On March 3, 1887, this teacher, Anne Sullivan, a graduate of Perkins Institution of the previous June, met Helen Keller for the first time.

When Anne Sullivan, later Mrs. Macy, went to Tuscumbia, Alabama, she took with her a doll dressed by Laura Bridgman, who was still living at the school, as the gift of the girls of Perkins. This doll became the subject of Helen's first lesson when the new teacher spelled the letters "d-o-l-l" into her hand in the manual alphabet. This, however, did not awaken a response and it was while holding her hand under water from a pump that the concept of word meaning penetrated the mind, and "w-a-t-e-r" was the first word that Helen Keller voluntarily spelled. Response to the underlying idea that finger positions represented the names of objects was evident in three weeks, and from there on Helen's onward march to heights of genius and greatness has been unimpeded.

To illustrate the development of methods used in teaching the deaf-blind, it might be well to tell of several children brought up in Perkins Institution, chiefly because their cases are better known, although there may be others equally successful in other lands or in other parts of this country. The first deaf-blind pupil to be taught articulation in the formative years of education was Willie Elizabeth Robin, who, in December 1890, when she was six, came to the Perkins Kindergarten from her home in Texas, "bereft of sight and hearing by severe illness called catarrhal fever," at the age of eighteen months.

Under a special teacher, Elizabeth's formal training began with objects—fan, hat, and ring—following the procedure established in the education of Laura Bridgman. She soon had a mental grasp of what was meant, and her response was so sure and quick that she achieved a knowledge of the objects within a fortnight. So steady was Elizabeth's progress that she received a diploma in June 1906, as well as a certificate for the completion of the full course in manual training. She was the first deaf-blind student to have been awarded a diploma signifying graduation from high school.

By way of contrast, insofar as background is concerned, consider Thomas Stringer. Born in Pittsburgh, Pennsylvania,

July 3, 1886, Tommy lost his sight and hearing through spinal meningitis when he was four years old. "A poor little waif of humanity," he entered Perkins April 6, 1891, described as "a mere lump of breathing clay." He showed intelligence, however, by creeping on all fours instead of walking and by moving backward rather than forward, having discovered that if obstacles were encountered it hurt less to hit his heels than to bump his head.

An affectionate little fellow, Tommy at first showed little interest in the objects given to him to feel until one day the teacher tried a piece of bread. This awakened an immediate response, perhaps because of the many times when Tommy had been hungry. It will be recalled that bread was suggested for objective teaching by the Spanish educator in his book published in 1795. Tommy grew to be an alert, honest young man who made up for his lack of advance in literary subjects by his competence in woodworking. With his fingers he could detect a bulge, crack, or irregularity that defied vision, and he learned to identify eight kinds of wood by the sense of smell alone.

Anna G. Fish, long associated with Perkins Institution, tells the story of how Tommy was given a block composed of two kinds of wood so skillfully joined together that no line of meeting could be felt. Asked what kind of wood it was, the lad smelled it on one side and then the other. Puzzled, he did the same thing over and over. At last deciding that this variety of wood was beyond his ken, he gave his impressions, absurd though he thought them to be. Pointing to one side, he spelled "pine," and for the other side, he spelled "white wood." When told that he had named them correctly, he was both pleased and relieved, and the persons who had put the pieces together to puzzle him were astonished.[5]

The continuous presence of deaf-blind pupils, from the admission of Laura Bridgman in 1837 to the present time, has focused attention on Perkins for its work with doubly handicapped children. Prior to 1931, there had been eighteen deaf-blind pupils in residence. In that year, a special department replaced the old plan of employing a teacher for each pupil.

Now teachers, skilled in speech building, are engaged only in classroom instruction, while attendants care for children outside of the classroom. In making this fundamental change, it is hoped to secure more skilled teachers on a professional level and by distributing responsibility to avoid both the loneliness of Laura Bridgman after her school work terminated and the lifelong dependence of Helen Keller upon first Mrs. Macy and later Miss Thompson.

The approach in general teaching was also changed from the method developed by Dr. Howe with Laura Bridgman. Instead of beginning with an object and having the pupil learn the name of it, a command is now the opening wedge. Most teachers begin with the command to bow. The beginning pupil places his fingers on the teacher's face, feeling both the vibrations of the muscles of articulation and the lip positions used in forming the elements of speech. The teacher will say "bow" distinctly, while she pushes the child's body into a bowing position. This is done again and again, until the muscular pattern of bowing is associated with the vibrations felt as the command is spoken. Often it takes months of daily work in short periods to get this idea into the child's mind and sometimes it is never accomplished. But after the first command is understood, the more complicated commands become progressively easier to teach.

Another vital change was to make speech the main medium of communication. Spelling in the hand was no longer taught those who could develop speech, and manual signs were not encouraged. The aim was to make communication as normal and natural as possible, so that anyone, not only those who knew the manual alphabet, could talk with the children. In earlier years, this was not thought possible, but now its practicality has been proved, and can be demonstrated by several accomplished students. The secret of the success of the new method is vibration, and it has become, in a large measure, sight and sound to the deaf-blind.

Building speech through vibration requires competent teaching. At first, the child has to be taught how to form his lips and place his tongue in order to make the fundamental sounds in somewhat the same way described by Deschamps in 1779. Beginning with "oo," "ah," and in some cases "ee," the child must learn to give these sounds in a natural voice, and then combine them into words as spoken by the teacher. It must be remembered that deaf-blind children are not naturally dumb. They are not able to imitate speech because they never have heard people talk—a principle first enunciated by Dr. Bulwer in his book published in 1648.

Taught to hear through vibration, the deaf-blind child must then build word meaning into the delicate varying vibrations of the throat muscles. He must then be taught to reproduce with his own vocal cords the sounds thus heard. This method was originally developed by Miss Sophia Alcorn, for many years a teacher of the deaf in the Detroit public schools, and modified considerably by Miss Inis B. Hall, the first head of the deaf-blind department at Perkins, and later, until her retirement in 1952, the first director of the department of the deaf-blind in the California School for the Blind.

To illustrate the progress possible under this method, consider Leonard Dowdy. Leonard came to Perkins in 1932 from Missouri. He lost his sight and hearing from spinal meningitis at the age of twenty-one months and had not learned to talk. When he came to Perkins, he was like a little animal, running about on all fours, and, displaying the same innate intelligence as Tommy Stringer, he had learned from experience that it was better to run backward than forward. A language study made of Leonard's progress at Perkins revealed that he learned to speak and to understand in his first year only forty words. In two years, he knew four hundred. Shortly thereafter, he was able to carry on a conversation with almost anyone, expressing ideas and doing the full work of the school in all departments.

While at Perkins, Leonard was a lively member of the community. Full of fun, he liked to be with other boys and was not above getting into considerable mischief. His acute sense of smell enabled him to distinguish people one from another. He also had an uncanny way of knowing whether a man or a woman entered the room. He made a mistake, however, during his first year, when a woman who had been smoking came to see him. On her arrival, he exclaimed, "A man." Since then, his knowledge has broadened and he now accepts the fact that women smoke. Flowers in a room, however, always confused him. Leonard also had an accurate sense of direction and is usually able to go to any place to which he has once been guided.

While Perkins Institution can claim a certain historic origin in successful work for the deaf-blind and over a century of continuous service, there are other places where the doubly handicapped have found help and instruction. The Nebraska School for the Blind has had a notable work with nine deaf-blind children, including Clarence Goddard, whose biography was published in 1926. The Pennsylvania Institution for the Instruction of the Blind, now called The Overbrook School for the Blind, has had several doubly handicapped pupils. In 1940, the New York Institute for the Education of the Blind erected a special building for the deaf-blind with unique facilities for their education, and from that time on has had a number of doubly handicapped pupils in residence. In 1943, the California School for the Blind opened a department, erected a building, and started a program under the direction of Miss Hall. Here deaf-blind children are being instructed successfully. Deaf-blind pupils have been received and taught in several other schools for the blind, notably Virginia, Indiana, Minnesota, Michigan, and Washington. In 1955, the Alabama School for the Deaf and Blind opened a special department for the deaf-blind.

Deaf-blind children have been educated in several schools for the deaf; in fact, at the beginning of the century there were more doubly handicapped children in schools for the deaf than for the blind. Kathryne Frick, whose autobiography was published in *The Atlantic Monthly* in 1930, attended the Pennsylvania Institution for the Deaf, and Helen May Martin, a gifted pianist, was a pupil of the school in Kansas. Ludivine Lachance was taught by the sisters in a school for the deaf in Montreal and Marie Huertin attended the Larnay Convent in France as a deaf-blind student. More recently, deaf-blind children have been educated in St. Mary's School for the Deaf in Buffalo, and in the state schools for the deaf in Michigan, Illinois, and Iowa, where a special department has been established.

At least two successful attempts to educate the deaf-blind were made in Europe soon after Charles Dickens had broadcast throughout the world Dr. Howe's achievement with Laura Bridgman. In Sweden, where a survey revealed a large number of deaf-blind children in the rural population, Madam Elizabeth Anrep-Nordin took a profound interest in their welfare. After securing the interest of the royal family, she secured legislative provision for their care. Coming to America, she visited several cities, spending a number of weeks at Perkins Institution. On her return to her home in Skara, Sweden, where her husband was principal of an institution for deaf-mutes, Madam Anrep-Nordin established a school for blind deaf-mutes, beginning with five pupils in 1886.

At approximately the same time, the Oral School for the Deaf in Hamar, Norway, admitted Ragnhild Kaata. Taught orally, she is conceded to be the first deaf-blind person to learn to speak. Both of these countries still carry on work for the deaf-blind, although in Norway that work is now assigned to the schools for the deaf, while in Sweden the deaf-blind are admitted to the school at Lund, where blind children with other disabilities are also accepted. In this school, where there were fifty children in 1952, all with blindness as a common handicap, the deaf-blind represent the smallest group.

England is following the Swedish plan, having a school for blind children with additional handicaps. This is at Condover Hall, and in 1952, 175 children were in residence, but only three were deaf-blind. A special teacher for the deaf-blind was trained in this field of education at Perkins Institution, and has returned to England. Australia and Greece have also sent teachers to this country for special training, the first to New York and the other to Perkins. France has two schools where deaf-blind pupils are admitted, one at Saint-Mandé for girls and one at Poitiers for boys. Because of the small number of doubly handicapped children in these schools and the variations in their abilities, the program is carried out almost entirely by individual instruction.

The German Republic also has two schools that accept the doubly handicapped, one at Potsdam-Bad, which is only for deaf-blind children, and the other at Stuttgart, where the deaf-blind children attend classes with the blind, but are trained separately in "writing into the hand." Switzerland cares for its deaf-blind children at the school at Chailly-Lausanne. Italy educates the doubly handicapped in a department annexed to the State School of Method in Rome, and Austria has a school at Graz, which "intends to dedicate its work to the training of deaf-blind children."

"Let it be remembered," wrote Helen Keller, "the deaf-blind children who are being taught will grow up. What are they going to do with their education and capabilities if there are no special friends trained to be the ears, eyes, and interpreters for them in the unpredictable vicissitudes of life?" [6] The answer to that question is not easy, but there are those who are seeking to find an answer.

No one has done more in this seeking than Peter J. Salmon, now head of the Industrial Home for the Blind in Brooklyn, which despite its name is one of the most modern sheltered shops for the employment of the blind in this country. In June 1945, Mr. Salmon opened a special department for the employment of the deaf-blind and appointed a supervisor to make every effort to gain the confidence and friendship of the doubly handicapped workers and to make their lives as happy and as normal as possible. There have been, and are now, deaf-blind persons employed in many of the sheltered shops for the blind. For many years, one was employed at the Perkins Workshop in South Boston. He was assigned to supervise the machine that picked apart the hair from old mattresses, because the noise that it made was so distracting to blind workers.

In 1946, the American Foundation for the Blind turned its interest to the deaf-blind and set up a new program known as the Helen Keller Department. The Department, under its own director, has become an active center for promoting interest in the doubly handicapped, and is endeavoring to list deaf-blind people and to analyze the services they need. It is also undertaking a program of public education, and through well-placed press and radio stories is doing much to focus attention on this small section of the blind population in this country, which has been described in the past as "the most neglected and the most handicapped in the world."

Until quite recently, all efforts for the education of deaf-blind children have been somewhat spasmodic and sometimes selfishly centered in the schools undertaking this work. For that reason, one of the most significant developments in this area was the Conference of Educators of Deaf-Blind Children, sponsored jointly by the American Foundation for the Blind and Perkins Institution, which was held at Perkins on April 13 and 14, 1953. The good response made by schools for the deaf was encouraging, for it indicated a revived interest in the doubly handicapped, or perhaps a greater readiness to tackle the problem.

The delegates present, after discussing the problems of educating deaf-blind children and the extreme difficulty of finding adequately trained teachers, recommended that a permanent national committee be established to deal with this matter. In September 1955, Perkins Institution opened a special class for training teachers of the deaf-blind to supplement its long-established courses for instructors of the blind. The Committee has also initiated plans to develop a program of research into the problems of the health and education of deaf-blind children. All in all, this looks like the most constructive action that has developed in this special field, and it certainly gives promise of a more hopeful future for the children of the silent night.

There is another area in the field of special education in which some constructive steps have recently been taken and where it is hoped final responsibility has been placed. This is with blind children who are too retarded for the normal school program or are definitely feeble-minded. While many feel that the ratio among the blind in these categories is high, mental testing proves that the number is not out of line with seeing children. Many residential schools are trying to aid their retarded pupils, for whom there often is no other source of help, through "opportunity" or special classes geared slower than the regular grades. These fall far short of the needs of this group, since few schools have the psychological or psychiatric aid that is essential for constructive work.

In 1921, Mrs. Jessie Royer-Greaves, distressed by the lack of progress being made by retarded children in the residential schools, resolved to give her whole thought and attention to a small group when she secured an old farmhouse with ample grounds in King of Prussia, Pennsylvania. Owing to her patient understanding of these doubly handicapped children, Mrs. Royer-Greaves accomplished wonders with her charges. But the farm school lacked the special facilities needed to do the job that cries to be done. Moving to an estate in Paoli in 1940, however, enabled a more effective program. The most recent attempt to meet this need with adequate buildings and outstanding services is the unit for the blind retarded opened at the Walter E. Fernald State School for the Feeble Minded at Waverley, Massachusetts.

At that school on September 13, 1954, the first complete academic year began in a $1,800,000 unit named after Ransom A. Greene, head of the Fernald School when the plans were being formulated. The new unit provided for approximately 250 patients with complete facilities for their physical and psychiatric care, education, training, and recreation. It is appropriate to have this new venture at the Fernald School, for the School had its origin in the old Perkins in South Boston and Dr. Howe was its head until 1880. While Dr. Howe might have granted that these deviate children should be institutionalized, he would not have liked having them segregated in a separate unit for both living and schooling. Both groups of children could certainly benefit by association, and friendships could be built up through the exchange of wits and sight. Many a sharp-eyed but dull-brained youth could get a therapeutic lift out of being eyes for one who has no sight. And vice versa.

But as Dr. Malcolm J. Farrell, superintendent of Fernald since 1945, said: "Just as 107 years ago the Commonwealth of Massachusetts answered the need for an institution for retarded children in an institution for the blind, so the Commonwealth today has answered the need for an institution to train the blind retarded in an institution for the retarded." [7] The significance of the Greene unit is that it has cast the die of responsibility for the retarded blind, placing it in a school for the retarded seeing. The danger of the Greene unit is that it may be filled up with mentally retarded adults, for the legislation placed no age limits on the beneficiaries and the children may become "blind of the second class," as were the pupils of Haüy's school in Paris when Napoleon in 1800 moved them in with the Crusaders in the Congregation of the Three Hundred.

8 FINGERS FOR EYES

As one surveys the early attempts to teach the blind, one cannot but be impressed by the prevalence of a single method—trial and error. There were no established ways nor indeed any tools of learning for those without sight. In common education, sight is the sense most used. It has been estimated that 85 percent of what is learned comes through vision. With that avenue of learning closed, there is need for imagination and ingenuity. And the story of how methods were developed and tools contrived is full of interest.

Trial and error may have played an important part in many of the first efforts, but the discovery of an effective medium of reading by the blind was sheer accident. Recall François Lesueur, the blind beggar whom Valentin Haüy persuaded to be his first pupil. For two years, Haüy and his pupil experimented with many ways of attacking their problem without success, and then Lesueur accidentally discovered that he could read the slightly embossed letters on the reverse side of a funeral notice fresh from the press. The fundamental importance of this accident was that it indicated to Haüy that the key to the education of the blind was the substitution of the sense of touch for the sense of sight.

Sensitive fingers, Haüy was convinced, could take the place of insensitive eyes, for as the blind teacher and psychologist, Pierre Villey, later wrote, "Sight is long-distance touch, with the sensation of colour added. Touch is near sight minus the sensation of colour, and with the sense of rugosity added. The two senses give us knowledge of the same order." [1] Even to this day, when a blind person wants to call attention to something that he is examining through touch, he will say, "Look at this," or if he wishes something that another has, "Let me see it, please."

There is, however, one definite limitation to the substitution of fingers for eyes and that is the extent of view. Eyes can see over a wide range and for long distances. Fingers can see only what they can touch and the horizon of the blind is thereby restricted to the reach of the arms. The blind man of Puiseau, when asked by the philosopher Diderot if he ever wished for sight, replied: "Were it not for curiosity, I would just as soon have long arms." In any consideration of methods and tools of learning, these two factors, the substitution of touch for sight and the restricted horizons, must never be overlooked.

With these sensory substitutions, experiments on the trial-and-error basis have been carried on from the earliest times. Early in the fourth century, the great scholar Didymus used an alphabet made of wooden blocks to further his education; and in the sixteenth century, Jerome Cardan, the Italian physician, astrologist, and mathematician, advocated the use of touch for the blind and a system of signs for teaching the deaf. Shortly after, there were two attempts to apply his principles. Francisco Lucas of Saragossa, Spain, carved letters on thin tablets of wood, the first recorded use of raised type for the blind; and Rampazetto, in Italy, incised letters on wooden tablets—both at about the same time, between 1575 and 1580, and both undoubtedly under the influence of Cardan.

In 1640, there is record that a French notary, Pierre Moreau, developed a system of movable letters cast in lead, and about the same time Udalrich Schönberger, in Prussia, employed letters made of tin. Georg Philipp Harsdorffer, of Nuremberg, Germany, in 1651 recommended wax-covered tablets on which letters could be written for the blind with a blunt-pointed instrument; and in 1676, Francesco Lana, an Italian Jesuit priest, proposed a cipher code based on a circle of dots enclosed in a square. He also advocated an arrangement of knots tied in strings. The talented French blind girl, Mélanie de Salignac, who made such a deep impression on

Diderot, was taught to read by means of letters cut out of cardboard, and to print with a pencil guided by a thin ruler. All of these were interesting attempts, but none was adequate for easy and facile reading.

Even before these trial-and-error experiments with forms of tangible type, other methods were explored. One of the earliest was the use of memory as a medium of learning. In Japan in the earliest days, memory was employed not only for the benefit of blind individuals, but also for the posterity of the nation. Instead of writing the history of the country in books, the accounts of important events were related to blind men who committed them to memory. The story was then passed on to younger men and thus transmitted from age to age with the greatest fidelity. The memory of the American historian, William H. Prescott, was phenomenal; in his older years he felt that he was failing because he could no longer retain in memory more than forty pages of copy. Memory was also used as the chief method of instruction in the early English schools. In 1833, one school reported that the inmates "had voluntarily committed to memory the whole of the Psalms contained in the *Book of Common Prayer*. This they have done," boasted the report, "in a shorter length of time than has been done in any similar institution."

Another early tool of learning was the string alphabet. Howe found this system used in the school in Edinburgh and brought one back to Perkins, where it now rests in the Museum. Various knots and loops in the string indicate the letters of the alphabet. Varying methods of this form of communication have persisted through the years. Villey reports that the blind musician Dumas wrote his music by means of pieces of cork, leather, and metal threaded on string. A mattress shop in this country for years used knots tied in strings for shop numbers and for instructions to its blind workers. A woman professor in an eastern college, not many years ago, when her sight began to fail, devised a system of reminders by differently shaped beads on string which she ran over just before giving her lectures. Dr. Enrique Rodriquez-Diago, of Barranquilla, Colombia, South America, is now advocating a system of communication, known as Cordellary, based on the Morse Code: a single knot tied on a string for the dot and a double knot for the dash. If, as is generally assumed, the string alphabet originated in Peru, this brings its practical use back to South America.

These forms of communication, however, could never become satisfactory mediums for reading. Reading implies the existence of books which contain ideas, descriptions, and dialogues expressed in words composed of letters and, in the case of the blind, letters that the fingers can read. That is what the early experimenters were seeking and what Valentin Haüy found through the chance discovery of François Lesueur. Through trial and error, Haüy sought to arrive at a tangible type that the fingers could easily read, but in doing this he fell into a serious error, for he was obsessed with the idea that a type suitable for the finger must also be pleasing to the eye. This became the guiding principle for all seeing people who, after Haüy, continued to develop types for the blind. In so doing, Pierre Villey said that the seeing "were talking to the fingers the language of the eye." [2] This, he maintained, was a fundamental psychological error.

Out of this error, a blind man was to lead the seeing. For at the same time that many new forms of line type pleasing to the eye were being promoted, a youth without sight, studying in the Valentin Haüy school, had the insight to find a way that would bring the language of the eye to the tips of the fingers. This development was not completely original, for it was based on a combination of raised dots that had been devised by a military man with full sight, Charles Barbier. He, however, was not concerned with the blind but was seeking a way to send along the battle line code messages that would be meaningless to the enemy and could be employed in darkness. He called it "night-writing."

Barbier, a cavalry officer attached to the French Signal Corps, had developed his system of dots and made his first report regarding it in 1808. Although acclaimed by the Academy of Sciences on several occasions, it did not impress the military authorities, and the system became something of a game among the people of Paris, who juggled the points around to see how many combinations could be made. In some unexplained way, Barbier brought his system to the Paris School for the Blind in 1820. It was given a trial by Dr. Sebastien Guillie, head of the School, to whom it seemed impractical, and it was officially discarded. A pupil in the school at the time, however, was impressed with the possibilities of the dot system and began to tinker with it. So successful was he in his adaptation of the point system of Barbier that it has become the accepted medium of reading and writing for the blind in all parts of the world and is known as braille.[3]

Louis Braille, the pupil in the Paris School, was born on January 4, 1809, in the little village of Coupvray, about twenty-six miles east of Paris. There were three other children in the family, living in an old stone house at the foot of the hill leading up to the village. The house was both home and shop, for in one part the father carried on his business as a harness-maker. The children had the run of the shop. Sometimes, they would hold the leather as their father cut long strips. At other times, they would sit at the bench playing at being harness-makers. One day, while handling his father's tools, Louis accidentally slit his eye with the harness-maker's knife. Infection soon spread to the other eye and in a short time all of his sight was gone.

It was a dark day in the household in Coupvray. To have a blind child was a great grief to the parents and like a death blow to the hope that they held for their bright youngest son. The accident, however, deepened the mother's affection for Louis, and the father took time to help him. Giving the little boy a stick, his father showed him the way to the well, and later guided him to a bridge nearby over a rapidly flowing stream. Louis loved to listen to the sound of the water rushing below, mingled with the vibrations of wagon wheels as they rolled over the bridge. Soon he was able to make his way up the hill to the village marketplace, which many years later would be known as Braille Square and would have in it a statue in his honor.

As soon as the little blind boy reached school age, he walked with his brothers and sisters to the village school, and soon surpassed his seeing schoolmates in learning. The father, realizing that he himself had not long to live, and anxious to assure the continued teaching and the security of his blind son, entered him in the National Institution for the Blind in Paris in February 1819. So proficient was young Braille at the school that, when his studies were completed, he was asked to remain, first as a junior instructor, and in 1828, at the age of twenty, he became a full professor, teaching history, geometry, and algebra.

Through his later years at the school, Louis' health was not good, although he continued to carry on with his teaching. When nearly forty, he was forced to give up many of his classes because of incessant coughing and his inability to make his voice heard during his lectures. When his illness became acute, Louis was taken back to the home village, where he died in the house where he was born at the early age of forty-three on January 16, 1852. Buried in the cemetery of Coupvray, his body remained there until the centennial of his death (1952) when it was exhumed and brought to Paris to rest among the immortals in the Pantheon. But the hand with the reading fingers was left to repose forever in the earth of his home town.

When Louis Braille undertook the adaptation of the Barbier system, he first determined that the cell of twelve dots, two vertical rows six dots high, was too tall to be comprehended by the finger. Barbier had made a stylus and slate for the writing of his system, quite similar to the ones used at the present time. Braille took one of the slates and soldered two strips across the frame, reducing the twelve dots to six, two vertical lines of three dots each. This brought the cell within the span of the fingertip.

Barbier's system was phonetic rather than alphabetic. Braille changed this by setting up sixty-three combinations of the six dots to represent the letters of the alphabet, certain common words, frequent combinations of letters, and musical terms. In making these adaptations, Braille was assisted by Alexandre Fournier, a former pupil of Valentin Haüy, who was then teaching in the Paris School. An early exposition of his new form of type is contained in a book on teaching music, written by Louis Braille in 1829, and embossed in the italic script of Valentin Haüy. Braille in this volume explains and illustrates his new system of point writing, including suggestions for contractions. While intended for ordinary writing, he states, its value for music, especially plain song, is pointed out. It was not, however, until 1834 that Braille had worked out in detail all of the possible combinations, including his musical notation.

Dr. Pignier, successor of Dr. Guillie at the Paris School, and the seeing teachers did not favor the new medium of reading, and forbade its use. The students, however, who were introduced to the system by Louis Braille in off hours, insisted upon using it, for here was a type pleasing and understandable to the fingers. In 1839, Braille issued a pamphlet describing in full the new system, giving due credit to Barbier for its origination, and to Fournier for his help in evolving the combinations. It was not, however, until 1854, two years after Braille's death, that the Braille system of dots became official in the school where it had been developed, and this occurred only when the students and the blind professors overwhelmed by their insistence the seeing members of the staff.

In advocating this new system of reading for the blind, Louis Braille stressed what he called "the principle of logical sequence." According to this, a line made up of the first ten letters of the alphabet, using the upper two rows of dots for symbols, forms the basis for succeeding rows. The second line, beginning with the eleventh letter, *k,* is an *a,* with the addition of the left-hand dot in the third row of the cell, and so on through *t.* The remaining letters of the alphabet, plus enough symbols to make the third row of ten, are formed by adding the two dots of the third line of the cell, and the fourth row is made by adding the lowest dot on the right-hand side of the cell. As the French alphabet contains no *w,* this letter was missing from Braille's original system. Introduced later to meet the needs of other languages, it is a *j* with the addition of the lowest right-hand dot of the cell.

No one is certain how Braille selected the combinations of dots for the first ten letters, or why he established the sequence of four lines. W. H. Illingworth, however, points out in explanation that it must be remembered that Louis Braille was, first of all, a musician, and that what he was originally seeking was a form of music notation that the blind could use in their employment as organists. He writes:

> This view would appear most reasonable, for it is more likely that the four lines had their origin in the requirement of the efficient representation of quaver, crotchet, minim and semibreve, than that a purely arbitrary arrangement of dots for an alphabet and some contractions should excellently and accidentally suit the necessities of musical notes . . .
>
> There are many variations of the Braille alphabet and contraction signs, but only one musical alphabet, and that practically as he made it, still unchanged, in all parts of the world where braille of every kind is used.[4]

Louis Braille undoubtedly had music in mind, as Illingworth claims, when he based his form of notation on the principle of logical sequence, but the fact remains that in his first announcement Braille places the writing of music as secondary and it is in its use for "ordinary writing" that the dot system soon superseded the line type developed by Valentin Haüy and won universal acceptance. But it was not without a struggle, not only between two systems, line and dot, but between two philosophies, one advocated by the seeing, that a type for the blind should be pleasing to the eye, and the other by the blind, who were interested only in securing a type legible to the finger.

Before the dot system reached England, books in line type were brought from France by Lady Elizabeth Lowther for the use of her blind son, Sir Charles Lowther. Securing similar type and with the help of a manservant, she printed in English a copy of the Gospel of St. Matthew. British schools, however, did not take kindly to the round italic type of the French, and attempts to improve it were soon under way.

In 1822, the Edinburgh Society of Art offered a prize, and in the following year a gold medal, for the best type for the blind. Six competed for the prize the first year and fifteen the second year. It is of interest to observe that, although conventional line type was the form generally in use, twelve of the fifteen competitors for the medal proposed arbitrary systems of forms or dots in place of letters. Despite the fact that the arbitrary systems outnumbered the line-type systems, the medal was awarded for a system of plain Roman capitals designed by Dr. Edmund Fry of London. This decision was based largely on the old fallacy that a suitable type for the blind must also be pleasing to the eye.

Stimulated by this award, the Glasgow Asylum for the Blind began to produce books in Fry's type under the leadership of John Alston, and they became widely used throughout Great Britain. There is record that at this time the "institution in Philadelphia wrote to congratulate him [Alston] on his system and to say that they had begun to turn out books according to his plan." On the strength of this, John Alston made an appeal for money to set up a permanent press, referring to the fact that books were being printed in America, and therefore the project in Scotland should "not be allowed to languish for want of money." Apparently he succeeded in raising enough money, for his press began to operate in January 1837, and in 1838 Alston is reported to have dispatched a large consignment of books across the Atlantic. By 1840 he had embossed all of the Scriptures.

Glasgow, however, was not to have the field to itself, for James Gall of Edinburgh, one of the competitors for the Edinburgh Society's medal, soon began to exploit his own form of type. This was an angular modification of the Roman letters, and in it Gall tried to combine the advantages of the ordinary Roman letter with an arbitrary system, but he failed to win the support of either side in the controversy, even though he claimed that his type was not merely the "best yet constructed for the blind, but the most perfect that can be." Gall, however, was a printer and therefore able to produce books without seeking financial support. Experiments were begun in 1834 and continued until 1838, when he published as his first book the Gospel of St. John.

A new form of type which, its exponents felt, would form a universal medium of reading for the blind was introduced in London in 1838 by Thomas M. Lucas, who had a school for blind children in Bristol. This type was later adopted by the London Society for Teaching the Blind to Read. In developing his type, Lucas used three forms: a straight line, a curve, and a dot. In combining these, he produced a system that was stenographic. Adherents to the Lucas system claimed that the shorthand features facilitated reading by the fingers, and told the story of a clergyman who, having been twelve years deprived of his sight, attempted in vain to read the common alphabetic type. Having acquired a knowledge of the Lucas stenographic system, he "now reads with such fluency as to perform his ministerial duties without any assistance, conducting two whole services every Sunday with the same ease and comfort as if he were not deprived of sight." [5]

In the same year that the Lucas type was introduced, another and even more arbitrary system was developed by a blind man named James Hatley Frere. His characters were neat and tangible, and although phonetic, differed from the Lucas system in that each word was embossed according to its pronunciation. An interesting innovation presented by Frere was that the fingers read the text from left to right on the first line, then dropped down to read the second line from right to left and so on. This was to prevent the skipping of lines. Although a society was formed to propagate the books, the project did not succeed, as the system proved to be too complicated.

One semiarbitrary type of raised letters developed during this period has survived. That is Moon type, named after its originator, Dr. William Moon. Born in Kent in 1880, Moon lost the sight of one eye through scarlet fever when he was four, and all of his vision by the time he was twenty-one. Financially well-to-do, he set out to explore ways of developing a form of reading that would be "open and clear to the touch." He did not resort entirely to arbitrary characters, but took the capitals of the Roman letters and reduced them to the simplest form. For example, the letter *A* was stripped of its crossbar and the letter *D* of its front vertical line. "Where I could not alter," Dr. Moon said, "or remove certain characteristics, I formed new characters." Nine simple characters set up in different formations resulted in an alphabet that was easy to read and also legible to the eye. In his printing, Dr. Moon followed the alternate-line reading system of Frere.

In 1847, the first book in Moon type appeared. Until the beginning of the twentieth century, all of the books promoted by the Moon Society, which the inventor started and supported, and which his children carried on until 1914, were devotional in character. In 1914, the Moon Society was taken over by the National Institute for the Blind, which still publishes a small number of volumes for that limited section of the blind population which prefers this form of simple type. Dr. Moon and his daughter Emily came to the United States in 1880, advocating his form of printing. Perhaps the most lasting result of the work of Dr. Moon and the Moon Society was the employment of people to teach the blind to read this form of type in their homes. This plan has developed into the present home-teaching scheme, and Dr. Moon is frequently referred to as the "father of home teaching."

When Dr. Moon died in 1894, books in his type were printed in 419 languages and dialects. And in many parts of the world today, there is still a demand for Moon books, especially among newly blinded persons who feel unable to master braille, and particularly from old people. With today's increased life expectancy, there may well be a revival of interest in this, the sole survivor of the old line types. Perhaps an indication of this was the starting up in 1933 of the production of Moon books for the first time in America by J. Robert Atkinson, founder of the Braille Institute of America in Los Angeles, California. For surely California is a haven of the aged!

The dot system was slow in reaching England, even though workers for the blind must have known of its use in the Paris school and of its official adoption in 1854. Yet in 1868, when Dr. Thomas Rhodes Armitage organized a company of blind persons and formed the British and Foreign Blind Association to put an end to the use of line types, he states: "There was not a single institution for the blind in the United Kingdom in which the Braille system was used, and the number of individuals who knew it probably did not exceed twenty." [6] Dr. Armitage, who was himself almost blind and a finger reader, took violent opposition to the prevailing principle that books for the blind should be legible to the eye as well as to the finger.

Opposed to all the line and semiarbitrary systems, Armitage became the most ardent advocate of the dot system of Louis Braille, even when many of his compatriots and most of the German teachers favored the more scientific form developed in the United States and later known as American Braille. When the first conference in Europe of teachers and friends of the blind convened at Vienna in 1873, Dr. Armitage was there pleading for the dot. Under his promotion and that of his association, the adoption of the Braille system was rapid. In 1879, the dot system of Louis Braille was adopted in Germany, where it had been strongly opposed on the ground that any arbitrary system would separate the blind from the seeing. In 1882, Dr. Armitage was able to report: "There is now probably no institution in the civilized world where Braille is not used except in some of those in North America." [7]

9 BATTLE OF THE TYPES

URNING to America, it is interesting to observe that somewhat the same pattern was followed in the selection of a suitable type for the blind as in Europe. Here also braille was accepted only after a long struggle. The first school to show any interest in this system was the one in Saint Louis in the late 1850's. Prior to this, however, there was much searching for a suitable type. Accepting the dogma of Haüy that type for the blind must also be legible to the eye, practically all developments were of the line type. The battle of the types in this country was at first waged between the promoters of various forms of line type. Later it was continued between the line types and the dot system, and when the dot finally triumphed, the battle went on between the advocates of several systems of dots.

One cannot but wonder whether or not this confusion, which caused the scrapping of three sets of plates for all the books for the blind in America, might have been avoided if, when Samuel Gridley Howe visited the Paris school, he had been more cordially received, and had been told of the young instructor than experimenting with a new form of type for the blind. Louis Braille had fully worked out his system of dots in 1834 so that, when Howe was there in 1832, he must have been struggling with the problem. If by any chance they had met, would not the discerning mind of the ardent young American have recognized the merit of the new system, and might he not have become a convert to the dot method? How different the battle of the types in America might have been if Howe had met Braille!

Earlier it was mentioned that John Alston, the Glasgow publisher of embossed books, had referred to the books being published in America, and that in 1838 a large consignment of his volumes had been dispatched across the Atlantic. These books apparently went to Philadelphia, for at the same time Mr. Julius R. Friedlander, head of the Philadelphia school, began to publish books embossed in practically the same characters as those of John Alston. These, however, were not the first books to be produced in the Philadelphia school, for in 1833 the first book embossed for the blind in America was produced by Jacob Snider, Jr., Recording Clerk of the Board of the Philadelphia school. Snider, according to the first annual report of that institution, "applied his mind to the contrivance of a method of printing for the blind . . . and happily succeeded." [1]

The Gospel according to St. Mark was produced, the report states, "in a style of unequaled typography for the sightless . . . and is an honor to this country, since it gives facility in this branch of instruction hitherto unattained here or in Europe." [2] Despite the high praise, this volume, which was produced in small Roman letters in upper and lower case, apparently did not succeed as happily as had been announced, for in 1834, when Mr. Snider offered to emboss on copper plates the Gospel according to St. John, the Board refused because of "no funds."

Another factor which may have had a bearing on this decision is that Mr. Friedlander was then getting ready to produce books in characters similar to those used in Glasgow, and for a time known as Philadelphia Type. Mr. Friedlander died in 1838, and not many books had emerged from the Philadelphia school under his auspices. In 1838, a school magazine in embossed type was inaugurated, the first of its kind in America, with the annual subscription placed at three dollars. Dr. Howe in his report for 1846 regretted that the press at the Philadelphia school had stopped "because it was making most important contributions for the library of the blind." [3]

When Dr. Howe returned in 1832 from his observation of

institutions in Europe, he brought back with him four books, which made up the first library of the Boston school. *The Gospel of St. John* and a small book on *Scripture Statements with Respect to Religious Doctrines and Moral Duties* were secured in Edinburgh. From York, England, Howe brought a book of raised diagrams to illustrate a contemporary school edition of Euclid, and in Paris he obtained the largest of the four books, one entitled *Extracts from the Best English Authors.* This last volume is believed to be the first book in the English language embossed for the use of the blind.

Printed in Paris in 1819, the *Extracts* was intended to help French students in their study of English. The implication in the title, "the Best English Authors," is hardly accurate because most of the stories are from the Orient or from Greece. They were, however, translated into the English language. The only extract from English literature is Brutus's speech taken from Shakespeare's *Julius Caesar.* All four of these books are still in the possession of Perkins Institution. They are embossed in three different forms of raised type and represent the starting point from which experiments in Boston began.

Early in his effort to educate the blind, Dr. Howe realized the importance of books for his pupils to read. He did not find satisfactory any of the forms of type in his original collection. He also made a careful study of the arbitrary systems that had been developed in Europe under the impetus of the Glasgow contests. His reaction to all was unfavorable, for, holding to the old fallacy that a type for the blind must be pleasing to the eye, he wrote: "Whatever merit they present, they labored under the great disadvantage of not being legible by the eye of common observers." [4]

Having eliminated any possibility of a type in arbitrary characters, Howe turned to the use of what he called "the common letter." The type that he developed was an angular modification of Roman letters in both upper and lower case. This became known as Boston Line Type and for over fifty years was the predominant print for the blind in the United States, and in 1851 a gold medal was awarded the exhibit of

Boston Line Type at the International Exhibition in London.

Having developed this form of type, Dr. Howe proceeded to build a suitable printing press. The first book to come from it was the *Acts of the Apostles* in 1835, then in 1836 the *New Testament,* and the *Old Testament* in 1843. Dr. Howe, however, proceeded immediately to print textbooks that were needed in his school, and especially atlases, which became one of Dr. Howe's original contributions to workable volumes for the fingers of his pupils. The trustees of the Institution apparently were not in full sympathy with the idea of entering into the business of printing and publishing, for the record shows that Dr. Howe had to secure support for his printing press outside of the school funds.

Apparently he persisted and was successful, for the press was soon producing more books than any other press in this country or in Europe, and, within several years of its establishment, volumes were being distributed in England, Ireland, and Holland, as well as to other schools in America. His volumes apparently reached far distant places, for in the files of Perkins there is a letter from a blind soldier in India telling of reading a copy of the *New Testament* which had reached that country. The success of the Perkins press was probably due to the fact that Dr. Howe's type was so compact that his books required only one-half as much space and could be printed for one-quarter of the cost of their European counterparts.

There is a good deal of evidence that the Boston press and the Philadelphia press, during its short period of existence, had a free exchange of books, both between themselves and with Europe. Early in this period, Dr. Howe made a plea to the institutions that were more or less competing in this limited field, suggesting that the presses get together and avoid duplicating books, which he considered an unnecessary waste. He took Mr. Alston of Glasgow to task for printing an edition of the Bible after one had been produced in Boston and copies sent to England. He felt that the amount of money spent in this duplication could have been used to the better advantage of the blind by having the Glasgow press produce some other needed volume, even though the types used differed slightly.

The difference in types, however, did not disturb Dr. Howe, for he stated, "The blind in the American schools read both kinds of print with facility, and it is not to be supposed that the blind of Britain have less cleverness than they." Even though there was a good free exchange of books between Boston and Philadelphia, both of these presses had difficulty in obtaining the same results from Glasgow. This, however, did not deter Dr. Howe from his determination to have all available books for his pupils, for he wrote, "We shall therefore proceed to purchase the books of the Glasgow press and put them into the hands of our pupils."

It is interesting to observe that in practically all presses, both in England and in this country, the first books to be embossed were portions of the Bible, and the highest objective was to produce the entire Scriptures. This indicates the religious motivation that was behind most of the work for those without sight, and one of the principal reasons for endowing presses and producing books was "that the Bible might be studied and that the blind by this means might be led from theological darkness into light." The American Bible Society paid for embossing the Scriptures in Boston Line Type in 1836, and later for the King James Version in braille and on Talking Book records. In 1953, it financed the recording of the Revised Standard Version of the New Testament. Indeed, religion still plays a strong part in the production of embossed books, especially magazines, for the great majority of periodicals for the blind today are sponsored by religious groups.

Dr. Howe did not share fully in this religious motivation, and early in his career, anxious to broaden the scope of reading material for the blind, he took steps to secure books from many secular sources. One of his efforts in this direction is of considerable interest, for in 1868 he wrote to Charles Dickens, who had visited Perkins in 1842, that "They [the blind] want something to gladden their hearts. They have had lugubrious food enough; they want happier views of life; they want some books which will give pleasure and joy in their dark chambers. . . . Your books do this, and I want the blind to have one of them at their fingers' ends." [5] Dickens responded generously to this request of Dr. Howe's, and, as a contribution to the blind of America, he arranged to send to Perkins Institution $1700 for the embossing of *The Old Curiosity Shop,* which was his own selection. It was embossed in Boston Line Type, and one of the original copies is still in Perkins Institution.

The Braille system of dots, slow in reaching America as in England, was introduced at the Missouri School for the Blind in Saint Louis in the late 1850's, by Dr. Simon Pollak, a member of the board who had observed its use in Europe. Dr. John T. Sibley, the head of the school at that time, opposed the dot system on the ground that it was arbitrary and not pleasing to the eye. In some way never divulged, the pupils secured information about the new form of type and as Louis Braille first promoted his form of writing "out of hours" so the pupils of the Missouri School surreptitiously employed the dot system to pass notes among themselves, to the utter confusion of their seeing teachers.

As in the Paris school, the blind pupils and teachers finally overcame the opposition of the sighted leaders, for the point system soon proved its worth, and in 1860 it was officially allowed. In 1862, the school reported that "great advantage has been derived from the use of the system of point writing known as Braille . . . but in music its excellency is especially manifest." The Board of Trustees, at a meeting held on June 30, 1863, credited the promotion of the new system to Henry Robyn, the head of the music department, and stated: "This Institution is the pioneer of the Braille system in this country, and Mr. Robyn certainly deserves the honorable title of benefactor of the blind." [6]

Although the French never sought to change the system devised by Braille, both the English and the Americans did. Typically, the Americans felt that they could even improve the system. One of the first to try was Superintendent William B. Wait of the New York Institute. Mr. Wait's conversion to the dot system resulted from a survey of 664 pupils in seven different institutions, all of whom used the Boston Line Type. His study revealed that out of this number, one-third were good readers, one-third read slowly by spelling out the words, and one-third failed entirely. A similar test was given to the pupils in the Missouri School where braille was used. This showed that two-thirds learned to read fluently, one-third by spelling, while none failed. This was enough for the energetic Mr. Wait. He swung to the dots, but determined to develop a better system.

Rejecting the principle of "logical sequence" which was the guiding force of Louis Braille, Wait developed the principle of "frequency of recurrence." This did away with the arbitrary arrangement of points used by Braille, and in its place Wait worked out a system whereby the smallest numbers of dots were assigned to letters most frequently used. The gain in this was that in reading or in writing fewer dots had to be distinguished, and, with the smaller numbers designating the most frequently used letters, there was considerably more open space on the embossed plate. This system became known as New York Point. Wait also discarded the six-cell unit of Braille and substituted a cell two dots high with a base of variable length. There is still some controversy as to whether this system was actually developed by Mr. Wait, for there is considerable evidence that Dr. Russ, the first principal of the New York Institute, had devised it, but certainly Mr. Wait promoted it with all his energy.

Michael Anagnos, the successor to Dr. Howe at Perkins, was reluctant to give up the Boston Line Type of his beloved father-in-law. He soon recognized, however, that the day of line type was over. Among the blind members of his staff were some who wanted to experiment with the dot system, and, with Mr. Anagnos' approval, Joel W. Smith, the blind head of the tuning department at Perkins and formerly a teacher in the Royal Normal College for the Blind in London, developed a system which was first known as "Modified Braille" and later called "American Braille." In his system,

Smith retained the original Braille cell, three dots high and two wide, but he adopted the New York principle of "frequency of recurrence."

This form of type is generally considered to have been the most scientifically arranged plan ever devised, and many of the old-timers feel that it might have been adopted in America and in fact in all the world if it had had as active a proponent as the New York Point had in the aggressive Mr. Wait. In 1879, Perkins adopted American Braille and in 1890 a small group of adherents known as the "rebel instructors" endorsed the system. Even in England, it was conceded,

> There is also a greater saving of time in writing as compared with the English Braille owing to the small number of dots required to be made . . . It is a matter of great regret that at the time the revision of braille in this country was in progress, advantage was not taken of the willingness of our American cousins to unite in the compromise in order to establish a universal system of braille.[7]

Because of the confusion occasioned by these skirmishes in the battle of the types, persons dependent on finger reading began to demand that action be taken leading to a uniform type. The first organized complaint came from a group of blind people who had gathered in Saint Louis in 1895 to form an organization which later, in 1905, became the American Association of Workers for the Blind. At its convention in 1901, a committee was appointed "to investigate various forms of tactile print and to labor for the adopting of some one universal system." In 1912, the Committee tested 1200 American and British blind and found that readers of British Braille made the better scores, but they also discovered weak spots in both systems. Acting on these findings, the Committee brought forth a new system, called "Standard Dot," but by its opponents "Standard Rot."

Since the time when Dr. Armitage eliminated the use of the line types in England (beginning in 1868) and when he threw his weight against a real consideration of American Braille, the British have never swerved from the six-dot cell devised by Louis Braille. They have, however, had many different ideas about the use of the dots, particularly in the combinations representing signs and contractions, that is, the use of a single symbol for a word or a combination of letters. These, however, were thrashed out by 1905, when a system called "Revised Braille" was announced. This consisted of three "grades": One, fully spelled words and no contractions; Two, a moderately contracted form; and Three, a highly contracted system, almost approaching shorthand.

The English Revised Braille found a more favorable reception in this country than the Standard Dot System of the American Committee received in England. This finally resulted in the abandonment of Standard Dot and the careful consideration of the adoption of Grade Two of the English system. Members of the American Committee, however, were not quite ready to go all the way in adopting Grade Two, for they were not willing to accept all of the English contractions. The Committee, however, did approve of forty-four of the English contractions, thirty-four of which were single symbols, usually the first letter of each word standing for the whole word, as for instance *k* for "knowledge," and ten were symbols representing commonly combined letters or part-word signs.

This resulted in a system that became known as Grade One and a Half, since it fell between Grade One and Grade Two of the British system. In 1916, this plan was recommended to the American Association of Instructors of the Blind and the following year to the American Association of Workers for the Blind. With the approval of the two Associations, Grade One and a Half, with its limited number of contractions, became the official system of braille in the United States.

At last it was thought that the English-speaking countries had a system of braille similar enough to be readable in both countries. But the hope was short-lived. The British refused to use Grade One and a Half because it added seven minutes to every hour of reading and required the fingers to trace over 11 percent more line lengths. The Americans, however, importing many books from England, soon found that the larger number of contractions was not as appalling as they had feared and that the assimilation of all the contractions of Grade Two was not too high a price to pay for a system which would embrace the English-speaking world.

Looking forward to that possibility, the American Association of Workers for the Blind, at their convention in 1923, dissolved the original Committee on Uniform Type and turned the whole matter over to the American Foundation for the Blind, which had been established in 1921. The Foundation wisely approached the problem by starting with a part on which it was easy to find common agreement. This was to settle upon a common system of music notation. Agreement in this area could be anticipated, since Louis Braille, when he adapted the system of Charles Barbier, referred to its value as a method of writing music.

Delegates from several countries attending a conference in Paris in 1929 soon agreed on an international standardization of the braille signs to be used in a musical code, which found universal acceptance. The conference, however, approved of three ways of using these signs. In this country, bar over bar; in England, bar by bar; and on the Continent, the paragraph style. A conference held in Paris in August 1954 failed to agree on a uniform style but laid groundwork for further consideration in 1956. The sole approach to unity since 1929 was in 1946 when Perkins Institution, which had held to the paragraph style, yielded and joined the rest of the American schools in common use of bar over bar.

Encouraged by the success in 1929 of this partial approach in the area of music to the larger problem and becoming cognizant of the leaning in the United States toward the English Grade Two, the American Committee again started conversations with the British authorities and reconsideration was given to the value of certain braille signs and contractions. The World Conference of Work for the Blind, held in New York in April 1931, proved an opportunity for representatives from many countries to talk over the diverse uses of the braille system. General principles were established at this conference and the details worked out in July 1932, when an American committee went to London where a final agreement was reached.

Under this agreement, the Americans adopted most of the contractions of British Grade Two, while the British gave up some of their contractions and accepted the reversal of the capital and italic signs. There were certain compromises in rules of writing that were also agreed upon, and with these adjustments Standard English Braille came into being. Both in England and America, this called for a gradual transition to the new form, books published in the old type being replaced as needed. In this way, the century-old battle between the English-speaking countries closed, and there is now full agreement and exchange of books.

While these developments were going on in Britain and the United States, other countries were having somewhat the same experience in trying to arrive at a uniform system of type for finger reading. Much of the difficulty, however, stemmed from many of the conflicts that have been described, except that only the dot system was involved, for in many cases, especially in the Far East, braille was introduced by missionaries from the West after the decline of line type. While the devising of a system of point writing for Japan is generously attributed to Kuriji Ishikawa, it is known that Robert Lilley, a Scotsman, reached Japan in 1875 and that he had a part in setting up a system which included the basic alphabet of the Japanese syllabary and many of its characters. In order to do this, it was necessary to extend the base of the braille cell from two to four dots. This form of braille continues in the land of Nippon.

A representative of the Scottish Bible Society, William Hill Murray, introduced braille in China after opening a school in Peking in 1876. In this, he was assisted by Mrs. A. Graham, daughter of Bailie Alston of Glasgow. To put the Northern Mandarin dialect into the dot system, Murray devised a form in which 408 sounds were represented. In 1910, the heads of the schools for the blind in China, in coöperation with representatives of the Scottish Bible Society, drew up the Union Mandarin System which became standard all over China. As the people in Canton, where Dr. Mary West Niles opened the Ming-sum School in 1889, did not use the Mandarin dialect, she put the Cantonese dialect into braille. This she ingeniously did by reducing through phonetics the many characters to seventy-two braille symbols. This system was later made the basis of the simplified language developed by Jimmie Yen in the attack on illiteracy in China.

India, perhaps, best illustrates how one of the Eastern countries has made a notable contribution to the solution of a common problem. When schools were first started in that country, each school adapted a braille code for the reading and writing of the dialect of the area that it served. At least ten braille codes have been in existence in India at one time, thus making it difficult to carry on uniform educational work and to enjoy the exchange of books. One of the earliest attempts to resolve this problem is described in the report prepared by the Rev. J. Knowles and Mr. L. Garthwaite and published in 1902 by the British and Foreign Bible Society. This outlined an ambitious scheme to provide a single braille code for all Eastern languages, called "Oriental Braille."

There were several other attempts to unify the codes, but nothing tangible was accomplished until 1942, when an expert committee of the Central Advisory Board of Education was appointed to draw up a uniform braille code. The code proposed by this committee was recommended for use in all institutions for the blind in India, but it was not generally accepted, and the controversy continued. In 1948, the government of India decided to review the question, and, in order to lift the matter from the arena of debate and to have it studied in an objective manner, the government requested UNESCO to initiate an exploratory survey of the question.

UNESCO accepted the responsibility and appointed as braille consultant Sir Clutha MacKenzie,[8] a distinguished blind veteran of World War I, who made a preliminary report of the world braille situation. The consultant and the committee of UNESCO felt that the matter was too broad to be confined to India alone, and in March 1950 UNESCO convened an International Braille Conference in Paris, which was attended by experts from the United Kingdom, the United States, France, India, Ceylon, Malaya, China, and Japan.

While a world braille was originally proposed, the conference felt that the matter would have to be divided up, and a separate code provided for each major linguistic area. The conference recommended the convening of three regional conferences, one for countries using the Arabic script, a second for countries using ideographic scripts, and the third for countries using Spanish Braille. The section dealing with the Arabic script has evolved for the first time a common braille code for that area, and work is progressing in the other areas.

A successful outcome is now assured, because UNESCO has set up and is prepared to sponsor the World Braille Council. In this undertaking, UNESCO is accepting guidance from the World Council for the Welfare of the Blind, organized in July 1951 and made up of representatives of over thirty nations. With this coöperation, there is every reason to believe that the battle of the types is over and that peaceful ways will be found leading to world-wide acceptance of braille.

1 0 MECHANIZING THE
DOTS

THE fundamental reason for the victory of the dot system over line type was the fact that, in addition to providing a more facile way of reading, it also proved to be a good medium for writing. None of the line types could be written. The attempts of Valentin Haüy to have his pupils write by pressing heavy pens over cardboard letters was a complete failure. John Alston's method of embossing Roman letters by using sharp pins placed in a frame pressed on paper, padded with flannel, was too clumsy to be effective. Picture Maria von Paradis with a cushion on her lap pricking out with a pin her letters to her blind friend Weissembourg, or William H. Prescott writing his scholarly histories on carbon paper with an ivory stylus.

All of these systems were slow, laborious, and unsatisfactory, and they were soon discarded, along with all the forms of line type except Moon. The dot system of Louis Braille lent itself readily to writing, and for this, the frame devised by Charles Barbier and reduced to half its size by Braille was an effective mechanical medium. Made like a folded hinge, the upper half has rows of oblong holes, the size of the braille cell, which form a matrix to guide the stylus used to punch the dots on a sheet of paper. This is done from right to left, for, to be read by the fingers, the sheet must be turned over. This may seem difficult to those who depend on sight, but to finger readers it is a skill readily acquired.

Braille as a medium of writing was further brought into popularity by the invention of a machine for the accurate and rapid embossing of the six-dot system. In fact, the development of the mechanical Braille Writer, somewhat resembling a typewriter, may have been the decisive factor in the battle in this country, for it turned the tide from the New York Point system to the orthodox braille. This device was invented by Frank H. Hall, who, in 1890, became the superintendent of the Illinois School for the Blind. Coming to the field of the blind from the public schools, he was appalled by the clumsiness of writing backward and the paucity of material for reading.

Hall immediately resolved to find ways to liberalize both of these mediums of learning, considered basic to one who had taught the sighted. He at once undertook a study of the various types. Hearing of the scientific aspects of American Braille, he visited Boston to inspect it and was favorably impressed. Hall then went to New York where Wait was able to win him over to New York Point. But when Hall began to develop a mechanical means of writing for the blind, he found that the variable base of New York Point did not lend itself to the even spacing required by the standard typewriter. The six-dot system of Louis Braille offered greater assurance of success, and, without further hesitation, the inventor shifted to that form of type.

Frank Haven Hall, whose contributions to the education of the blind have hardly received adequate recognition, was born in Mechanic Falls, Maine, on February 9, 1841. After serving in the Twenty-third Regiment, Maine Volunteer Infantry, in the Civil War, he taught for two years in Towle Academy. In 1866, Mr. Hall went to Illinois, and there he remained until his death in Aurora on January 3, 1911. In that state, he was considered "the greatest pedagogue in Illinois in his day." His tenure of office as Superintendent of the Illinois School for the Blind in Jacksonville extended from 1890 to 1902, with an interlude of four years, 1893–1897. The interruption and his short career may be explained by Edward E. Allen's reference to Mr. Hall as an outstanding contributor to the education of the blind and a "martyr to the American spoils system; a prophet unhonored in his own country."

Hall completed his Braille Writer in May 1892. This was a small, compact machine with a moving carriage similar to that of the typewriter and with provision for standard-sized sheets of paper to be inserted for embossing. A letter was embossed on the paper through the simultaneous pressure of the appropriate keys at one stroke, three keys on the left side and three on the right side, corresponding to the two vertical rows of three dots each in the braille cell. This machine was accepted with great enthusiasm, for it provided a convenient, accurate, and reasonably easy method of mechanical writing for the blind.

The successful development of a braille writer, however, did not come right out of the clear. Prior to 1892, there were many attempts to secure a good writing device for the blind. On January 7, 1714, a patent was granted by Queen Anne for a device "for the impressing or transcribing of letters singly or progressively one after another as in writing, whereby all writing whatsoever may be engrossed on paper or parchment so neat and exact as not to be distinguished from print." The applicant for the patent was Henry Mill, an English engineer, who announced his device as an aid for the blind. There is considerable doubt whether Mill ever completed a model measuring up to the ideal set.

More than a century later, between 1845 and 1850, William Hughes, a worker in the field of the blind in England, made a device called the Typhlograph for the head of the School for the Blind in Manchester. Intended originally for embossing letters, it was subsequently modified to make impressions through carbon paper, embodying a principle now common in the latest model of Varityper.

Perhaps the first machine that proved to be adequate for practical use was one made for Maria Theresa von Paradis, the brilliant blind musician of Vienna, called a Schreibsetzgerat. It was developed by a mechanic named Wolfgang von Kempelen, of Pressburg, Austria, in 1799. The last known working model of this machine was destroyed in the bombing of the Blindiana Library and Museum in Vienna during World War II. Two early reports of writing machines made for the blind come from Italy. In 1808, an inventor, Turridi di Castelnuovo, made one for the use of the blind daughter of a friend, and in 1856 Guiseppe Ravizza, a lawyer, developed a device in which he introduced a ribbon inking system.

In France, there was early interest in a mechanical means of embossing letters for the blind to read. In 1784, a machine, the first that embodied the manual keyboard, was invented in Marseilles by M. Pingeron. In that same city, a printer, Xavier Progin, was the first to use the type bar in a machine which he developed in 1833. In 1837, while Louis Braille was still experimenting with his system of dots, another blind teacher in the Paris School, Pierre Foucault, was tinkering with a device that employed radial rods to emboss letters. His objective was to bridge the gap between writing for the seeing and for the blind which he feared would be created if the arbitrary system of dots came into common use. Later, Foucault developed a machine that embossed a cuneiformlike letter so effectively that it attracted wide attention when exhibited at the International Exhibition held in Paris in 1855.

In the United States, the first patent for a device designated for writing for the blind was granted by President Jackson in 1829 to William Austin Burt. Called a Typographer, it introduced the method of paper feeding carried over in later machines, but there is no record of its success. Among the first of the many others seeking to perfect a mechanical writing device for the blind, was Charles Thurber, of Worcester, Massachusetts, who in 1843 constructed a machine and applied for a patent. This was the first machine with a movable carriage. There is evidence that Thurber tried to interest Dr. Howe at Perkins, for there is a specimen of his printing in the files dated August 1844, which states that the machine is "operated by keys like a piano." This machine was never perfected for practical use. In 1845 Thurber patented a second machine; this was not a typewriter but was intended to perform the motions of the hand in writing.

In 1856, another development for imprinting embossed letters for the blind was patented by Albert Ely Beach, an editor of *The Scientific American*. His machine introduced the basketlike disposition of type bars and type. Although it worked, its operation was slow, and its practicality restricted, because it embossed the letters on tape rather than on sheets of paper, a system later used in the Banks braille writer, produced about 1940. Beach did introduce a new feature: the embossed copy was in full view of the writer, which later proved its worth for sighted typists.

In 1860, C. Lotham Sholes, of Milwaukee, was urged to turn his attention from working on a device for paging a bound book to one that would write mechanically. Benefiting by the earlier experiments made in seeking a writing device for the blind, Sholes, associated with Samuel W. Soule and Carlos Glidden, both of whom were printers, worked for seven years and finally produced and had patented in 1867 a working model. The first machine was a primitive combination of under-strike type bars, operated by keys similar to those on a piano keyboard.

Thomas A. Edison, working at the time on a device to transmit letters of the alphabet over telegraph wires, invited Sholes to bring his model to Newark, New Jersey, and made many suggestions toward its perfection. The inventors called their device a typewriter, the first appearance of that term. Offered to the Remington Arms Company at Ilion, New York, for production, it became the first successful commercial typewriter when put on sale in 1876 as No. 1 Remington. In 1897, the Underwood No. 1 typewriter was put on sale. This featured visible writing as developed by Franz Wagner, found in Beach's model, and now common to all writing machines.

Out of these many experiments seeking to fulfill the objective set forth in the patent granted by Queen Anne, there came not a writing device for the blind but the modern typewriter, the fundamental machine of present business enterprise and an essential tool of all who write. Mark Twain was the first author to submit a typewritten manuscript to a publisher. This was his book, *Life on the Mississippi*. Even as the telephone was the result of Alexander Graham Bell's search for a hearing aid for his deaf wife, the typewriter is the outcome of research for a device for the blind.

The blind, however, did not lose thereby, for in an advertisement of the Sholes and Glidden writer published in 1875 is stated, "This machine is a great boon to the blind. They can soon learn to write with it. The attention of the teachers of the blind is especially invited." This proved to be true, for today the commercial typewriter is as essential to the blind student as the Braille Writer, as its use is taught in all schools for the blind, and for the benefit of seeing teachers more written work is done on typewriters than on braillers.

Mr. Beach in announcing his earlier machine, had prophesied that the fair sex would be ideal operators. And so it has happened, for hundreds of well-qualified blind typists and transcribers are finding employment in the business world, and indeed, the copy for this chapter was dictated and was transcribed by such a well-trained typist. From typists without sight has come the now universal touch system, for it did not take long for the office manager to realize that if a blind person can use a typewriter, surely a sighted typist can gain time by keeping her eyes on her copy and not on her fingers.

Incidentally, another effort to find a medium of writing for the blind resulted in a convenience for the seeing. A book published in Paris in 1800 describes in detail a proposed fountain pen for the blind and in 1806 a German named Müller actually made a hollow pen which could be filled with ink so heavy that, after writing and drying, it left a line sufficiently raised for the fingers to read. The heavy ink gummed up the pen so that it seemed at the time not feasible for its intended purpose, but later, by using a free-flowing ink, it became the modern fountain pen. In an effort to overcome the ink problem of the early pen, a blind person, Richard Dufton, invented a so-called ball-point pen, which he held to be far superior to an ink-holding pen, and which is only now coming into its own.

In the meantime there was a continued interest among the blind to devise a machine for point writing. One of the most interesting was that developed in 1865 by Joel W. Smith, originator of American Braille. Called the Daisy Writer because of the six petallike levers clustered in the center that operated the six dots of the braille cell, Smith's writer was a compact device which embossed the desired symbols on paper lying flat on a hand slate when the right combination of petals was pressed. This was undoubtedly the first successful mechanical device for writing braille in the United States. However, it lacked the sturdiness and effective ease of writing which Mr. Hall attained by his adaptation of typewriter construction.

The Hall Braille Writer, after its introduction in 1892, evolved through a number of changes that increased its efficiency, but the fundamental principle remained the same. Mr. Wait of New York, not ready to accept defeat, invented in 1894 a machine called the Kleidograph that could handle his system of type. In 1910, the Howe Memorial Press of Perkins developed a braille writer on the Hall principle with an improved paper feed; and, in 1931, another model that provided a back spacer. Similar machines, notably the Stainsby-Wayne in England and the Picht in Germany, were later developed and are widely used in Europe. The American Foundation for the Blind introduced in 1933 a more elaborate type of braille writer made by the L. C. Smith Typewriter Company. This incorporated many features of the commercial typewriter.

In 1950, the Howe Press offered a model built on entirely original principles. This machine eliminates the overhanging carriage, has an arrangement that controls the pressure so that all dots are evenly embossed, and has a unique paper holder. So impressed were the officers of the American Foundation for the Blind with the preliminary models of this new writer that in 1947 they shared with the Howe Press the costs of the tooling necessary for production in large quantities. In 1954 the Royal National Institute for the Blind in England adopted the model developed at Perkins. The Perkins Brailler is proving to be a very adequate machine for braille writing and is acquiring universal use.

When Frank H. Hall had produced his machine to speed up the writing of braille, he turned his attention toward overcoming the paucity of reading material for the blind which he had decried. He soon discovered that this could be accomplished by the adaptation of his principle of writing to the production of machine-punched plates from which books could be speedily embossed. Changing the hand-operated writer to a foot-powered machine placed on a large standing frame of great strength, Hall developed a device that would with the same fidelity and facility emboss metal plates. Placed on a press, either rotary or platen, pages of embossed books for the blind could then be run off from the plates in any quantity. Mr. Hall's first Braille Stereotyper, as it is called, was shown at the Chicago Columbian Exhibition in 1893, where it attracted wide attention. Schools immediately secured stereotypers to produce plates, even though many used hand-operated wringers for their printing.

It should be on record, however, that Mr. Hall's stereotyper did not originate the production of books embossed in braille. His device facilitated a speedier and more efficient way for their embossing. Prior to his time, there were some books—not many, it is true—set up either from metal slugs using braille systems or from plates hand punched. One blind man in England, John Ford, between the years 1872 and 1885, made by hand all the plates for the embossing of the Bible. In doing this, his hammer struck the punch making the required dots over two million blows. The first real printing press for the blind in the United States was invented and operated by Henry Robyn, head of the music department in the Missouri School for the Blind, in 1865. In this, he used metal slugs each carrying a braille symbol. These were set by hand, locked in a frame, and placed on a flat press, and the pages were embossed by the pressure of a soft-faced roller.

Braille books, printed as they were at first on one side of the sheet, made bulky volumes. For example, the Bible printed in that way would make a pile of books so high that the reader would need a stepladder to reach the top volume. Soon an inventive mind learned how to operate the stereotyper so that the line on one side alternated with the line on the reverse side. With more precise instruments, it later became possible to adjust the embossing so that the points on one side fell between those on the other, and thus the space required was cut almost in half.

Although the late Edward E. Allen reported that he had a stereotyper operator, Frank C. Bryan, who printed by interpoint in 1898 and there is record of similar embossing in England in 1900, the credit for its introduction into the United States is generally given to the late Walter G. Holmes. After observing it in England in 1912, Holmes tried out this principle in the *Matilda Ziegler Magazine,* which he edited. The first books to be published in interpoint appeared in 1926: *Closed Doors* for school use by the Howe Memorial Press, and the *Dawn of a Tomorrow* by the Braille Institute of America in Los Angeles.

With the development of the stereotyper and the later electrification of this mechanical means of embossing, and the use of the interpoint system, fast-running presses soon began to produce books for the blind in great quantity. With the increased production of braille books, the problem of size loomed larger. Experiments are now being made in England for the use of plastic dots instead of embossed, which may be one solution. These dots can be applied to paper much thinner than that now required to enable embossed dots to stand up under the pressure of finger reading. This is called "solid-dot braille."

An entirely new way of reducing the bulk of braille and one that offers also a unique means of reading is being developed by the International Business Machines Corporation. The material is punched out on tape and placed in a small device. The tape raises braille dots on a reading surface as it passes through the machine. The present tape rolls would take one-third the space required for embossed books and IBM hopes to reduce this to one-twelfth. The reading machine obviates the need for bound volumes and is in itself a clever and useful device.

The first books for the blind in the United States were

embossed by the schools, each of which had its own hand printers. As the process was slow and expensive, the supply was meager. As early as 1836, Dr. Howe tried to secure federal funds for books for the blind. While on a trip to Ohio in 1837, he went to Washington and petitioned the Congress to establish a library for the blind, but in this he was not successful. Again in 1846, he suggested that the seven institutions for the blind then in existence "send a deputation of their pupils to Washington for the purpose of giving an exhibition before the members of Congress and enlisting their feelings; and that a petition should then be presented asking for a grant of money or land that would yield at least $100,000."

Again Howe was ahead of his time, for it was not until 1879 that the Congress allocated bonds yielding $10,000 a year for books for the blind. These books, however, were not for general distribution, but were restricted to the use of the existing schools for blind children. Later this was enlarged to include appliances and the amount of income was increased to $125,000 a year. To administer this grant, the American Printing House for the Blind was established in Louisville, Kentucky, three years after the death of Dr. Howe.

Selection of Kentucky as the center for printing was due to the fact that in Louisville a national nonprofit institution designed to manufacture and provide embossed books and tangible apparatus for the blind at cost had been created by a charter granted by the Commonwealth of Kentucky on January 23, 1858. Prior to that, however, and two years after the death of Dr. Howe, his successor, Michael Anagnos, raised a fund sufficient to endow a printing press in memory of his predecessor. Known as the Howe Memorial Press, it has published embossed books and manufactured appliances for the blind from that time until the present day.

Four other printing presses for the blind have more recently been established: Clovernook at Cincinnati, Ohio, in 1903; the Ziegler Press in Monsey, New York, in 1907; the Braille Institute of America in Los Angeles in 1919; and the National Braille Press in Boston in 1927. The presses in

Monsey and Boston restrict their work almost entirely to the publication of certain magazines for the blind. The other two share, with the Howe Press and the American Printing House, in the production of books for the Library of Congress.

To provide books for the adult blind, Congress was approached in 1930 and through the Pratt-Smoot Bill, enacted on March 3, 1931, a project "to provide readers with a wealth of literature hitherto unavailable" was set up. The original grant in 1931 was $100,000, all of which had to be spent for embossed books. In legislation approved August 8, 1946, the grant was increased to $1,125,000 annually, $200,000 of which must be spent for embossed books and the balance for recorded books and Talking Book machines, a medium of reading for the blind introduced in 1934. This legislation was amended July 2, 1952 to permit the use of this reading material by children.

The administration of this project was placed under the Library of Congress because, as far back as the time of the Spanish-American War, John Russell Young, then librarian, started to collect all possible books for the blind, stating that "a special library of the blind would go far toward the complete idea of a national library." At that time, the Library of Congress had a collection of books for the blind totaling under 25,000. They were in several forms of the dot system, plus some books in Moon type. Since 1932, when Standard English Braille was adopted, all books for the adult blind under the Pratt-Smoot Bill have been embossed in Grade Two, which means that there is now uniformity.

Possibly the best way to show the growth and extent of reading matter for the blind in the United States, both by finger and by ear through Talking Books, is to report that on June 30, 1955 there were available for reading 1,373,286 volumes, of which 980,374 are in braille and 58,324 in Moon type, and there were 334,588 containers of Talking Book records holding over 4,000,000 disks. This total, however, represents but 7,480 titles—4,316 in braille, 2,773 recorded, and 391 in Moon type. There are also available a considerable number of books that have been hand embossed by volunteer transcribers.

During the calendar year 1954, 194,607 volumes in raised type and 1,111,383 Talking Books were mailed free from 28 regional libraries to 52,357 readers. Since 1904 it has been possible to circulate books for the blind through the United States mails free of postage. This special service has been extended to other countries. At the Conference of Educators of Blind Youth held in Bussum, Holland, in the summer of 1952, Colonel E. A. Baker, President of the World Council for the Welfare of the Blind, announced that the Postal Union had granted free postage for embossed literature and material for the blind passing through the country where it originated, the countries through which the mail may pass, and the country of destination.

Truly great progress has been made, when it is recalled that one hundred years ago, braille was not known anywhere in the world except within the little group concerned with its adaptation in the Paris school. A century and a quarter ago, when work for the blind in the United States was first undertaken, there were but five books in this country, the *Gospel According to St. Mark,* printed in Philadelphia, and the four books brought by Dr. Howe from Europe to Boston, all of which are now museum pieces.

11 EARS FOR FINGERS

OOKS for finger reading, while a great boon for the blind for over a century, have always taxed nervous energy and presented physical problems for persons whose fingertips lacked the essential sensitivity. In 1932, the American Foundation for the Blind began to investigate the extent of these reading difficulties. On the basis of returns from libraries circulating embossed books, it was revealed, according to the Foundation, that less than 20 percent of the blind people of the United States read with their fingers with sufficient facility to enable them to make fullest use of the braille library books then available. "As a matter of fact," the report stated, "not more than 10 percent of the blind have ever mastered finger reading well enough to enjoy embossed books."

While there is a bit of suspicion that these statistics were somewhat slanted for propaganda purposes, efforts were soon initiated to resolve the difficulties revealed in the investigation. These led to the determination to employ in reading the sense of hearing, thereby using as the substitute for eyes, ears instead of fingers. The possibility of this substitution goes back to the first recording of the human voice on a wax cylinder by Thomas A. Edison.

It is said that Edison, when applying for a patent on his talking machine in 1877, predicted its use for the benefit of the blind. It was, however, many years before this evolved. Ironically, the first step was the use of Dictaphone records in the early day classes for blind children in Cleveland and Minneapolis. More recently the Ediphone has been used both in classrooms and in offices, the Soundscriber has been the means of producing reading material, and recorders, both wire and tape, have become almost standard equipment for a blind person, especially college students. In the meantime many blind people found pleasure in the phonograph and all enjoy the radio.

Ear reading of recorded material really became practical for the blind through the development of the long-playing disk. In this transition the American Foundation for the Blind blazed the trail. As a medium of ear reading, a special type of phonograph disk revolving at $33\frac{1}{3}$ revolutions per minute, instead of the then prevailing 78, was developed. Cut at a pitch of 150 grooves a minute, a twelve-inch record provided on each side sixteen minutes of reading. For the use of these records 20,000 reproducers were built as a WPA project. In 1934 the first records and reproducers were ready and were named "Talking Books."

Even before this the British had become interested in recorded reading for the blind, chiefly through the leadership of Sir Ian Fraser, chairman of St. Dunstan's, center for the war blinded, and a governor of the British Broadcasting Corporation. Difficulty with getting sufficient reading matter on a single disk caused Sir Ian to abandon the idea, although he is now interested in a wider international use of this medium of reading for the blind. Later the National Institute for the Blind developed a record which, revolving at 24 revolutions per minute, makes possible twenty-five minutes of reading on each side of a disk. The newest machines in both countries are now standardized to play at $33\frac{1}{3}$ revolutions per minute, thereby making possible the exchange of records. Leaders in other countries are now turning from disks to tape using commercial recorders. To provide multiple copies a studio to duplicate master tapes in any language is being set up in Paris by the American Foundation for Overseas Blind.

More effective ways of reading by the sightless are being sought through experimental work now in progress. The present objective of researchers is to skip embossing, the medium of finger reading, and the present system of recording for ear reading, and to make available the contents of ink-print books through tones simulating the human voice. During World War II, under the high stimulus of war activity and the freer use of money for research, new ways to accomplish this objective were explored.

Early in the war, the National Research Council appointed a Committee on Sensory Devices, under the able leadership of Dr. George W. Corner, of the Carnegie Institution of Washington. The return of blinded soldiers and the new findings in such fields as radar and electronics made many feel that modern science could do something for the blind. This Committee promoted work in several areas, but in the field of the blind it first became concerned over the possibility of developing a way of reading that would be easier than braille and thereby make available a wider selection of books. Its ultimate aim was to find a means of opening directly to the sightless the same publications used by the sighted.

The basic medium of accomplishing this has been available since 1873, when Willoughby Smith of England discovered that the electric resistance of selenium is influenced by light. Almost immediately this principle was applied to the universal problem of securing a medium of reading for the blind. In 1874 a Frenchman, Ernest Recordon, presented at the Paris school a device called l'Electro-lecteur, which activated through electrical impulses sixty-four needles and receptors capable of embossing on paper ink-print letters. At the school Recordon tried to relate his device to the writing machine that Alexandre Fournier, associated with Braille in the development of the dot system of writing, had devised. L'Electro-lecteur was demonstrated at the Congress of Blind Schools held in Vienna in 1875.

In 1879 another Frenchman, Camille Grin, using selenium cells to scan printed material, completed a device for reading through the sense of touch, called the Anocaloscope. After an abeyance of a score of years the idea came up again in England, where after ten years of experimentation Dr. E. E. Fornier d'Albe of London introduced a device called the Exploring Optophone. This was originally intended as a general aid to the blind in finding their way about by detecting light. When light from doors and windows fell on the photoelectric cells, it caused buzzing sounds in earphones worn by the user.

The principle that enables light to be reported through photoelectric cells, on which the Exploring Optophone was developed, was further adapted by Barr and Stroud, Ltd., of Glasgow, in an effort to produce a reading device. In doing this, the engineers sought to get from patterns of black and white the same response as from darkness and light. This led to what was called the black-reading Optophone. A printed book placed face down on a glass plate was moved over a series of five cells. As these scanned a line of type, white caused no response, but when the black print of a letter was encountered it was transposed into sound according to its shape. Each of the five cells reported with a different tone, ranging from a high note for the top cell down to a low note for the bottom one.

These varying tones indicated the shape of the letters. For example, a lower case *l* would be reported by the four upper tones sounding simultaneously, a lower case *h* would have the same four tones followed by the tones of the three middle notes, and a *p* would be reported by the four lower tones followed by the three center tones. The promoters of the reading device did not claim that the identity of the individual letters could be readily recognized, but their report stated "when the alphabet has been learned, the motif for each letter is recognized as a whole and later in the reader's practice the more extended motifs for syllables and even words will become familiar." [1]

Two of these machines were brought to the United States in December 1922, and a number of studies were set up to test their practicality. The report of these studies indicated that the highest reading speed attained was fifteen words a minute, although the literature of the manufacturer stated that a woman in England read twenty-seven words a minute. Mechanically, the machine was satisfactory, and it fulfilled the principle desired, but as a practical medium of ear reading for blind persons, it could not compete with finger-reading braille.

At the World Conference of Work for the Blind held in 1931 in New York, another device using photoelectric cells was demonstrated by Robert E. Naumburg of Cambridge, Massachusetts. Extensive tests of it were later made at Perkins Institution. Instead of transposing the printed word into sound, Mr. Naumburg proposed to reproduce it in raised line type on a sheet of aluminum foil. When a page of a book was placed face down on the printing Visagraph, as this machine was called, an electric eye scanned the ink print and picked up the black formations of the letters. These were passed through a whirling disk and transformed into electric currents operating five magnets. The magnets actuated printing bars which embossed upward on the aluminum foil the letters that were being scanned. Reproduced in large type, the horizontal lines of the letters were solid, while the vertical portions were dots. For reading, the fingers ran over the letters raised on the aluminum foil.

During World War II, the Committee on Sensory Devices called in Mr. Naumburg as consultant, and, following his principle, a much smaller and more refined device of this type was developed, but its accomplishments did not greatly exceed the earlier tests and the expense involved did not justify quantity production. In 1955, new interest in the Visagraph was aroused when it was reported that through an old German process print letters may be pin-pricked inexpensively on old newspapers and are adequate for a single reading.

The Committee on Sensory Devices felt more hopeful about the reading method demonstrated on the Optophone and took steps to refine the instrument and improve the process. The development of this work was assigned to the Haskins Laboratories in New York, and placed under the direction of Dr. Paul H. Zahl, with Franklin S. Cooper in charge of engineering. From the engineering point of view, tremendous gains were made. The old Optophone, about as big as an office desk, was reduced to a size about half-way between an electric razor and a fountain pen. The resulting new device, engineered by the Radio Corporation of America, reported the printed material scanned through a system of audible signals. Because of its size, it was called the Electronic Pencil.

Despite the refinement in size and some improvement in the clearness of the sounds reported, a number of tests, especially the very scientific approach to the problem by the Institute of Human Adjustment at the University of Michigan, revealed that results were not so good as those attained on the old Optophone, and ear reading by means of the Electronic Pencil did not by any means approach the speed considered desirable. In short, as Dr. Corner wrote: "The instrument is able to gather and transmit all the information necessary to depict a letter to the ear. It is the human ear and the auditory connections of the brain that cannot easily convert the pattern of warbled sound into recognition of letters and words. The auditory system was evolved for different functions." [2]

The difficulties involved in what are called "direct translation aids," which convert the visual letter into patterns of sound or touch, with a rough resemblance to the original letters, led to concentration on a second type, generally known as a "recognition device." The function of this type of appliance is to identify printed letters and transform standardized patterns of them into sounds simulating the pronunciation of words. It is hardly to be expected that the best of machines could reproduce exactly the spoken word, particularly in English where so many words have two pronunciations as well as dual meanings. What results is an entirely new language which sounds like speech in an unknown tongue, although it does resemble English in length and meaning of the words and in grammatical construction.

The Haskins Laboratories carried on considerable research to determine the factors affecting the ease and intelligibility of auditory signals, with special emphasis on speechlike sounds. This involved the use of two appliances: the Sound Spectrograph, which analyzes the complex tones of the spoken material and presents the results as black-and-white patterns, and an instrument that converts patterns into corresponding sounds, called a playback. The Spectrograph was based largely on the principle developed by the Bell Telephone Laboratories in their analysis of human speech, but differs in several ways to meet differing needs. It does, however, fulfill the first objective of effectively transposing spoken words into patterns, but the development of a satisfactory pattern playback was delayed by difficulties involved in the transformation of the patterns into intelligible sounds. When this project was discontinued by the termination of the Committee on Sensory Devices at the close of the war, a grant from the Kellogg Foundation enabled Mr. Cooper to continue the work. He developed a playback to the point where recognizable sounds can be produced, but it has never been put into production.

In other laboratories in this country and in England, the search for a reading device for the blind continues. At the Research Laboratory of Electronics, Massachusetts Institute of Technology, Dr. Clifford M. Witcher, a noted physicist who himself is without sight, has been doing research on several aspects of visual prosthesis. While primarily interested in the development of guidance devices, Witcher is giving considerable thought to ways of mechanizing reading for the blind. In this area, he claims that the main problem is that of the redundancy of the printed word and of finding ways to reduce it. C. E. Shannon, of the Bell Telephone Laboratories, has estimated that printed English is about 70 percent redundant, whereas Witcher claims that Grade II braille has a redundancy of 67 percent.

A device for ear reading, therefore, must have the ability to cut down not only the redundancy of the printed word, but also better the lesser redundancy of braille, if it is ever to become an acceptable substitute for finger reading. And that, claims Dr. Witcher, "constitutes the basis on which communication theory can contribute most to the visual prosthesis problem." [3] What Dr. Witcher is expressing technically is that the scanning of ink print produces an overloading of the sensory channels through high redundancy, which, while it does not hinder the eye in reading, does slow down comprehension by ear. For that reason, all of the devices previously described, based on the principle of direct translation, have failed. On none could more than thirty words a minute be read, and that is not good enough to be a substitute even for finger reading.

Dr. Witcher and other researchers hope to overcome this problem through improved recognition devices. Perhaps the most successful instrument of this type is that of Professor David H. Shepard of the Intelligent Machines Research Corporation, Arlington, Virginia, which he calls an Analyzing Reader. This is a departure from the old method of more or less photographing the letters as printed, which was not only slow but also led to confusion when different type faces were employed. Dr. Shepard, in his analyzing of ink print, uses the electronic-computer approach. By this method shapes are analyzed in terms of their linear relations and converted into letter signals which are reproduced in tones that are understandable. The technology of this process is now well defined. All that is needed is financial support to put into production a recognition device that gives promise of serving as a successful reader for the blind. The unit cost of such an aid has been estimated to be about the same as that of an average home television set.

Another attempt to reduce redundancy, and in this case of the spoken word rather than print, is through a device that in a way telescopes speech. Such a device has been developed at the University of Illinois by Dr. Grant Fairbanks. This he calls a Time Compressor, because its purpose is to compress the time that it takes a person to speak a certain number of words at the normal rate. As a professor of speech, he has attacked the problem from the point of view of phonetics and speech values. Dr. Fairbanks began his experimentation by snipping the tape on which the verbal material to be compressed was recorded, thereby taking out what proved to be unessential elements. In the final device, this condensing is done electronically. When played back, the intelligibility of the recorded speech depends upon the degree of compression.

In tests, it has been learned that, when compressed 10 percent the reproduced speech seems the same as normal speaking; when compressed 25 percent, it sounds like Danny Kaye, but is still understandable to most listeners; while at 50-percent compression it is difficult for many to understand clearly the output. The problem now is to ascertain to what extent normal human speech may be compressed and still be understood. This has been estimated at a minimum of 20 to 25 percent. While this may sound a bit difficult to accept by all but the scientifically minded, it is surprising how effectively, through experience and with concentration, the human ear can learn to hear and to interpret strange sounds. To a skilled engineer, the slightest unusual purr of a motor means trouble, and how often fond mothers cannot understand why the gurgling of their offspring, so full of meaning to them, is not accepted as proof of the baby's ability to talk.

While most of this developmental work is aimed at speeding communication in the commercial field, the Time Compressor may be a boon to the blind ear reader.. Readers of Talking Books, especially the recently blinded, often become irked or tired by the time factor of ear reading compared with eye reading. For that reason, many are demanding that Talking Books be speeded up. Pupils in schools for the blind often jump the speed of reproducers from the specified $33\frac{1}{3}$ to 45 revolutions per minute. This makes faster reading but it raises the pitch to a point annoying to sensitive ears. The Time Compressor may be the means of resolving this aspect of ear reading. The hope that workers for the blind have for it is that it may increase the amount of reading that can be recorded on present disks and still be intelligible to ear readers.

Another field of activity that the Committee on Sensory Devices entered early was the search for and development of an efficient guidance device. In this area the first substitute for the eye was the ear, but more recently there has been a shift to the fingers, a reversal of the change in seeking a substitute for sight in reading. The fact that through the use of radar ships can locate obstacles in the dark and that planes can land through a fog made people feel that the same principles ought to be applied to a device to enable blinded servicemen to walk with certainty down a city street or to find their way in country lanes. Probably in no field of research have so many forms of aid been proposed. These have ranged from appliances too heavy and cumbersome to carry to minute ônes attached to ordinary spectacles. Early in this study, Dr. Corner pointed out that it must be remembered that "radar, wonderful as it is, can only pick up and transmit visible patterns. Somebody with good eyes must watch the screen where the images are formed."

The chief problem in designing a guidance device is to present to the blind person patterns that permit him to make decisions as would a seeing person in the same situations. The Exploring Optophone of 1912 failed as a guiding device because the indication of light might be the reflection of sunlight on a concrete wall rather than the signal for a clear road ahead. This led to a search for a form of energy that could make this distinction and be able to report obstacles. The possibilities of attaining this objective through the use of supersonic energy, ultraviolet rays, and visible light were all explored. Most of the early efforts were centered on the use of supersonic energy and ultraviolet rays, although what is now felt to be most promising is a device using direct light.

In 1944, the Committee entered into a contract with the Haskins Laboratories in New York City to act as a center for testing the several devices and to provide a technical staff to interpret the findings. The Committee first made a survey of the travel needs of the blind and concluded that two objectives should be sought: first, the development of a short-range obstacle locater that would report objects within a range of ten feet; and second, a recognition device that would give a plan-impression effective enough to identify objects and present a mental construction of an unseen environment.

A number of corporations with experience in related fields coöperated in attempts to produce devices to fulfill these objectives.

The Brush Development Company of Cleveland worked on an appliance using a crystal-type electronic generator; the Hoover Company of North Canton, Ohio, adapting some of the principles used in silent carpet cleaners, undertook to produce a device in which supersonic pulses were generated by mechanically struck bars; the Stromberg-Carlson Company of Rochester, New York, long engaged in studies in acoustics, did extensive fundamental research on the physical characteristics of supersonic energy and developed a visual aid using a magnetostriction type of generator; and the Franklin Institute of Philadelphia attempted the design of an instrument using ultraviolet light. In the meantime, the United States Army Signal Corps, in the Evans Signal Laboratory at Belmar, New Jersey, had independently started on the development of a device using visible light as the medium of detecting objects.

The value and practicality of these devices were explored in various places and a wide variety of reactions were recorded. In general, it may be said that many of the early engineering difficulties were resolved but that the human factor proved to be more difficult to standardize. The early problems presented by the Exploring Optophone, which reflected light regardless of substance, were largely overcome by the Signal Corps through a technical procedure known as modulation. A more difficult problem met in all the devices was that, although they could detect the rising of the curb across the street, they could not report the drop of the nearer curb. This, however, has now been overcome by a special device known as a curb detector developed by Dr. Witcher at M. I. T.

Steps are now being taken to combine the curb detector with the Signal Corps device, the effective use of which is being tested at Haverford College, under a grant from the Veterans Administration, by Professor Thomas A. Benham, another able physicist without sight. At first it was thought that the Witcher curb detector and the Benham obstacle finder could be put "in the same box," but, at this writing, Witcher is trying to produce a complete travel aid that will include both objectives and Benham is seeking to extend the range finding of his device and to include an effective step-down detector. He writes with optimism, "There is every expectation of success and satisfactory results. . . . The help of many and the application of much diligence is a far better basis for hope of a successful conclusion to the research in this field." [4]

Of all the devices that have been developed so far, regardless of the energy band used, only two have successfully reached beyond the narrow-beam or simple probe type—the British clicker device which generates high-frequency sound pulses and reports the reflections heard from obstacles on each side of a path, and the optical aid developed at the Haskins Laboratories which, through automatic scanning, provides recognition of simple objects at a distance. The other devices have restricted their objectives to a simple reporting of obstacles in the path directly ahead, although, to receive information in a larger arc, any of them may be swung from side to side.

All of these travel aids are portable instruments, one model resembling a large flashlight and another a motion-picture camera. They are carried by the blind person so that the beam of energy strikes the ground about ten feet ahead. Information is obtained by the reflection of the beam of light or supersonic waves from an obstacle that may be in the way. Early in the research, attempts to recognize larger areas were given up but more recently the objective has been to obtain reports that indicate: (1) the outer region with an "awareness" signal, (2) the middle region with an "attention" signal, and (3) an obstacle with an "avoidance" signal, which indicates that the blind person had better alter his path if he wants to avoid the obstacle.

One of the significant decisions during the many trials was to change the signal reporting an obstacle from an audible buzzing, indicating by its intensity the closeness of the object, to a tactile report either through vibrations or electrical impulses incorporated in the handle of the unit. Benham has successfully developed such a system in the Signal Corps device. This change was made mandatory by two factors revealed in the trials: first, it was difficult to hear sound reports in traffic or where there was considerable outside noise; and second, it enabled the use, for supplementary reporting, of the natural sense of obstacles that so many blind persons develop, and in which hearing is a primary factor.

The innate sense of obstacles which some blind people develop to a point where they do not need or want a mechanical travel aid is one of the chief reasons why the machines have met with a lukewarm reception on the part of many sightless persons. There are also others who still prefer to rely on the most ancient of guidance devices, the cane. This, too, has felt the refining influences of science. From the tall staffs seen in ancient pictures of blind mendicants, it has swung to the well-known white cane or, for the more sensitive, to one resembling a fashionable walking stick. During World War II, the use of the cane was developed into a definite technique through the work of Dr. Richard E. Hoover at the Valley Forge General Hospital, a center for the war blinded. In this development, the cane was lengthened to about half-way between the staff and the walking stick in order to give a scanning range of five feet. A procedure for integrating the swing of the cane with the natural body movement was developed and is now part of the training course for pupils in many schools for the blind and in the rehabilitation of newly blinded adults.

There is another widely known method of mobility for the blind. This is through the use of guide dogs, a method as old as blind mendicants. There are very early reports of the use of dogs in China and a more modern record of their possible use in Austria when in 1819 Johann Wilhelm Klein, the educator in Vienna, described a method of training guide dogs in his book on the education of the blind. It was not, however, until World War I that dogs were especially trained for guidance of the blind. Toward the close of that conflict, the German government trained dogs for soldiers and sailors who had lost their sight in the war, and so successful were they that the service was extended to civilians. In 1924, Mrs. Harrison Eustis, an American with kennels in Switzerland, having observed the work in Germany, began experimental breeding with German shepherd dogs which she had been training for patrolling the Swiss border and for finding lost persons. Articles in the *Saturday Evening Post* in 1927 brought information to the United States, and Morris S. Frank of Tennessee applied for a dog to serve him as a guide.

Mr. Frank went to Switzerland to receive his dog "Buddy," and Mrs. Eustis was persuaded to come to this country to set up a training center. Since 1930, The Seeing Eye, Inc., has operated in Morristown, New Jersey, and a quarter of a century later more than 2000 dogs are serving their blind owners. It takes three months to train a dog and a month to teach dog and owner to work together. The success of this form of mobility depends on a careful liaison between animal and human and for that reason careful selection must be made of persons who can use dogs. It has been estimated that less than 10 percent of the blind in this country can benefit by guide dogs because of temperamental relations. Dogs, especially trained, are now widely used in many European countries, and training centers in this country have been set up in Michigan, New York, and California.

One more area of activity on the part of the Committee on Sensory Devices should be included, for while it was intended for the partially sighted, it is proving helpful to persons whose visual loss falls within the legal definition of blindness. This is the effort to make ink-print books readable by visually handicapped persons through magnification. The Committee sponsored a study of the problem by the Dartmouth Eye Institute under E. J. Ellenbrock, which also produced two magnifiers capable of enlarging ordinary book print, through direct lens magnification, to the size of 18- and 24-point type, the sizes used in Sight-Saving Classes for partially seeing children.

In the meantime, Herbert Jahle, working in the Physics

Department at Harvard University, developed a device which magnified five and twenty-five times by projection. This device was at first about the size of two telephone booths. In an attempt to simplify and to reduce in size this form of magnification, G. Farrell, Jr., at Perkins Institution, produced a pilot model about the size of a shoe box. To study the problems involved in reading through magnification the Committee authorized a study by Perkins Institution. This was conducted under the able leadership of Professor Walter F. Dearborn, Director of the Psychoeducational Clinic of Harvard University.

Further development of the use of magnification as an aid to the visually handicapped was undertaken by the Franklin Institute of Philadelphia. Through a grant from the Kellogg Foundation, both Jahle and Farrell worked for a time on these developments at the Franklin Institute under the direction of Frank Cooper. This research resulted in a reasonably compact instrument which magnifies any printed text six times and is now in limited production. At about the same time, the American Foundation for the Blind began work on a smaller projection device based on the principle of the reproducer of microfilm. Called the Megascope, it is now serving many people with limited vision. One of the significant discoveries in this area of research was that people with vision as restricted as 5/200 could use such aids, provided they had been taught print letters, which makes such aids of great value to persons with failing sight.

The ability to read ink print by persons well within the present definition of blindness would seem to complete the cycle from eyes to fingers, fingers to ears, and, through magnification, back to the eyes. And while this has been achieved largely by science, there is still a human factor which must not be overlooked. For as Dr. Corner, Chairman of the Committee on Sensory Devices, pointed out in his final report, "It is too much to expect that any of the . . . devices will ever be a comprehensive substitute for vision in performing the activities which it is intended to aid. We may, however, expect that some, and possibly all, of them will be helpful in certain specific tasks." [5] From the engineering point of view, great progress has been made, and workers for the blind must always be grateful to the stimulus to investigation that the urgency of the war effort provided.

On the other hand, the essential human factor, especially in handicapped people, must never be ignored, and the danger of overloading the blind with cumbersome devices must be avoided. The development of scientifically perfect contrivances is today relatively simple. It is more difficult to take the measure of the human spirit of the visually handicapped which causes them to want to succeed on their own. And yet, as Dr. Corner has written,

The hopeful advances of civilization must be seized and turned against the ancient disabilities. The young science of psychology offers its gift of self-understanding . . . Modern physical science and engineering also have aid to offer, and those who know the electron and those who understand something of the infinitely more complex human personality and nervous system must cooperate to apply this knowledge to the problems of the sightless. [6]

12 COMPENSATION— THE EARLY OBJEC- TIVE

ALTHOUGH the first constructive efforts to alleviate the lot of the blind in response to the challenge of Rousseau were for children, there is early record of grave concern for sightless adults. This was especially true of beggars who, seeking alms, roamed the countryside and cluttered the streets of nearly all the countries of Europe and Asia. Although begging was earlier tolerated both as a means for the sightless to eke out a living and as a medium of merit for the givers, enlightened social conscience and religious impulse were reacting against the dire condition of the segment of society whose blindness was in large measure no fault of their own.

History abounds in early efforts to alleviate their lot. Inspired by Christian charity, their objective was to shield helpless blind men and women from the world through shelters and asylums. Such was the intention of Saint Lymnaeus, who, in the fifth century, established a refuge in Syria. Here the hermit saint gathered the blind and built for them, adjoining his hermitage, special cottages, where he taught them to sing pious songs; but, it is interesting to note, he permitted them to accept alms from those who were moved by their singing.

A century before this, the spirit of religious charity motivated many to want to help the handicapped, particularly the blind. Saint Basil, who became Bishop of Caesarea in A.D. 370, was particularly zealous in gathering handicapped persons of all types into the monastic institutions that he controlled. For each disabled group, he provided separate quarters, but all engaged in common work and worship. They were instructed in the faith of the Church, for Bishop Basil, it is said, had equal zeal in seeking converts. Here the blind found refuge from the world and shared in the kindly ministrations of the Bishop's sister, who, wrote Gregory, "was eyes to the blind, feet to the lame, a mother to orphans."

In the seventh century, Saint Bernard, Bishop of Le Mans, founded an institution in the northwest of France, into which he gathered the blind from the highways and byways and taught them to chant the Church's liturgy in the stately tones of Gregorian plainsong. And in Japan, when Prince Hitoyaso became blind in 871, he gathered the sightless in his palace in Kyoto, and under the patronage of later emperors they received many benefits. Through guilds in which they were organized, the fields of music and massage were reserved for the sightless of Japan. In Egypt in 970, the University of Al-Ashar opened its doors to the blind, offering a twelve-year course. Because there was no printing system for the blind at that time, all lessons were memorized.

In Europe, it was not until 1254 that an effective organized effort to help the blind was made. In that year, Louis IX is said to have enlarged L'Hôpital des Quinze-Vingts, close to the Rue St. Honoré in Paris, in order to provide a home for 300 crusaders who had lost their sight while held as hostages for the king, who had been captured by the Saracens in 1250—twenty being blinded each day for fifteen days until the ransom arrived and the king was released. The truth of this story is now questioned, but there is evidence that a shelter for the blind was already in existence at the time and that, in 1254, the king bought the property and built a new house. This he opened to blind crusaders, who were parading the streets of Paris asking for alms and crying "Sainte Terre, Sainte Terre," indicating that they had lost their sight in the Holy Land.

The king gave to the blind crusaders an allowance from his privy purse on condition that they make soup for the poor.

He also bestowed upon the "congregation of the three hundred" distinct privileges, such as freedom from taxation, the right of asylum, and the privilege of wearing a distinctive garb. The inmates held daily services and in return for gifts said masses for the repose of the souls of the wealthy. It became fashionable for the powerful and the rich to visit the Quinze-Vingts and to bestow gifts upon it. In time, the institution itself became wealthy and lost its high purposes.

In 1777, the house provided by Louis IX was sold to Louis XVI for enlargement of the Royal Palace, and the pensioners were moved to quarters in the old barracks of the Black Musketeers on the Rue du Charenton. Here they fell into dissolute ways and roved the streets of Paris as beggars. The blind men who took part in the burlesque at Saint Ovide's Café which so moved Valentin Haüy came from the Quinze-Vingts. And here, to the distress of Haüy, his first pupil, François Lesueur, sought refuge in his later years.

The Quinze-Vingts has survived to the present day and visitors to Paris interested in the blind still visit it. But it has settled down after its long and turbulent history and now fulfills its original intent of providing a home for 300 blind men and their wives. Its importance lies in the fact that it early set the pattern for the asylum care of the blind, a plan that was followed in many countries in Europe. In Chartres, the Six-Vingts was founded, but it never equaled its prototype in activity or prestige. Its inmates were chiefly known for their activities in making trouble for the pilgrims visiting the Cathedral, and in the seventeenth century the Six-Vingts lost its identity by merging with a hospital.

Most of the early asylums for the blind were merely attempts to take the itinerant sightless off the streets, and little was done toward training them for integration with or living among the seeing. The asylums were merely palliatives and did not meet the real problem that arose in the Middle Ages when beggary became rampant. During that time, the blind changed from pathetic, but appealing, persons, pleading for alms because of their affliction, to pests on the roadsides and nuisances at all public gatherings.

In this transition, which began in the fourteenth century and culminated in the sixteenth, the blind may well have had a case. For they were the victims of occupational modernization. The sightless bards had lost their livelihood with the introduction of printing and the production of books and news sheets. Blind mendicants, because of the changed attitude toward them, were not getting the same return from their former profitable and comfortable locations at the city gates and the temple doors, and they were seeking redress.

In Spain, the sightless acquired the sole right to sing in public places, a privilege they held until the Revolution of 1868. In the north of Italy, the blind, utilizing the medium of their demotion had their songs printed and sold them as they sang on the city streets and country waysides. In Portugal in 1749, in another effort to offset the loss of employment through the growing preference for printed matter, the blind were given the exclusive rights to sell newspapers and songs on the street. In all these efforts of redress, the blind soon found that to succeed they had to organize.

In China and Russia, blind mendicants early learned to work in bands. They held congresses, elected leaders, and assigned areas for begging. As early as 1377, a guild of blind persons was organized in Padua, Italy, following a pattern established among the artisans of that day. Called "Fragila," the guild regulated the places and conditions of begging, the chief occupation of its members. The guild also adopted measures for mutual protection, prohibited the "stealing" of guides by one blind person from another, set penalties for members who cursed (perhaps those who didn't give enough!), and ordered all members to report incidents of cursing. The guild required all blind persons to be members and set up a system of pensions. It is known that in 1616 this guild had 1500 members, owned five pieces of property (presumably homes for the aged blind), and sent four representatives to the governing body of the city.

In 1661, a guild was formed in Palermo, Sicily. Sustained by an annual grant provided by sympathetic citizens, this group secured permission in 1690 to use as a meeting place

a hall owned by the Jesuits. The blind brotherhood was
governed by its own officers: a superior with two "cojuncts"
and six "consultators." Made up mostly of musicians and
singers, the guild finally developed into a sort of musical
academy where new songs were composed. Every member was
under obligation to submit a new poem in praise of the
Virgin to the congregation on the eighth of December. Audiences were assured because Archbishop Mormile granted
an indulgence of forty days to any person who would listen to
a blind man recite a spiritual poem.

One of the significant social consequences of the early
"congregations" was that it gave the blind a realization of
their own strength when bound together. No longer were
they content with the simpler forms of help provided for
the blind from religious motivation, be it Christian or Moslem, and, with no training for self-help, blind paupers began
to demand from society and from the Church the right to
exist on a higher economic level.

The Reformation created a social crisis for the blind because until then the Church had been largely the source of
relief. Many of the asylums were closed and new ways to help
had to be found. This proved to be a turning point, for the
new ways were motivated chiefly by a desire not to take beggars off the streets but to bring relief to all defective and
needy persons, including the blind. Out of this movement
emerged a social conscience expressed in civic support of
the needy and secular provision for defectives. As the problem was more acute in the cities, the first "poor ordinances"
developed there.

As early as 1437, Frankfurt-am-Main had established poor
relief; from 1450, the city officials of Cologne distributed
alms; and in Antwerp, after 1458, there was a "Master of the
Poor." These were forward steps, but it was not until the
next century that the new reform spirit promoted ordinances
that were more constructive. Notable were those enacted in
1522 in Nuremberg, which specified that all needy persons
should be supplied with food, and the ordinance in Strass-

bourg, adopted the following year, which provided for every poor person a weekly dole according to his need.

It soon became necessary to carry the same methods into rural areas. This called for action by the state and was accomplished through the adoption of the so-called "chest ordinances," which sought to revive the old churchly care of the poor with considerable civic control. Under the new plan, the money available for poor relief from both Church and state was pooled. Institutions were opened under secular rather than religious auspices, especially in Germany. In that country in 1531, Emperor Charles V imposed on every community the responsibility of feeding its poor. But if the means were not sufficient, needy individuals were entitled to go out and beg.

In 1748, it was decreed in Prussia that in every district the magistrate, in coöperation with the pastor, must create a poor chest. Laws passed in Austria in 1754 and in 1787 gave to every citizen of a given community or one who had resided there for ten years the right of relief in case of need. In France, the care of the poor remained under church control until the Revolution, although as early as 1254 Louis IX had decreed that all parishes should keep a register of the poor and undertake measures for their relief.

Countries untouched by the Reformation also began to reorganize their care for the poor, under government rather than religious auspices. The New Ordinance of the city of Ypres was a most notable example. It was based on a study of the poor made for the city of Bruges entitled *On the Subvention of the Poor* and published in 1526. This struck a new note in the care of the blind, for it maintained that they should not be allowed to sit around unemployed but should be put at some useful employment as a contribution toward their support.

In England also, the state took over the work for the needy that had been conducted by the Church before religious and monastic properties were confiscated. In 1573, a tax was levied on real property for the care of those unable to work.

In 1601, Queen Elizabeth I had a law enacted that required the justice of the peace in every parish to appoint from two to four respected citizens to serve as overseers of the poor and to have authority for a tax to be levied on the parishioners for the relief of the old, the sick, the blind, and the crippled poor. This still stands as the basic law of all poor-relief work in England as well as in America.

Long before this legislation, there had developed in England considerable voluntary help for the blind, which grew in strength and continues to the present time. The earliest attempt to offer such voluntary succor to the blind in England was in 1329 when a London mercer, William Elsing, opened an asylum to give shelter to 100 men near the London Wall. This was known as the Elsing Spital. It was confiscated during the Reformation, as all hospitals of the Middle Ages were considered religious foundations. Henry de Gower, Bishop of Saint David's, who died in 1347, founded an asylum at Swansea which he liberally endowed with his own funds, as well as with the revenues of three parish churches.

Charitable concern for needy blind individuals early expressed itself in gifts and bequests designated for pensions. It is interesting to observe that many of these contributions were given to the old City Companies for administration. The earliest of these is the Worshipful Company of Paint Stainers, incorporated by Edward VI in 1469, to which through the years large sums of money have been left for the blind. At the present time, the Company grants to 200 blind persons pensions of £10 a year, while the Clothmakers Company distributes each year £12,000 from funds given to it since its founding in 1528. Other City Companies providing pensions for the blind are the Drapers, the Cordwainers, and the Goldsmiths. The last was founded in 1813, the others prior to that date.

An interesting illustration of the objectives in those days of transition is found in the creation of the first institution for the blind in Scotland. In 1793, David Johnston, an energetic divine of Leith, founded the Edinburgh Asylum. Its exact title was The Society for the Relief of the Indigent Blind. In a couple of months, workshops were opened and the title was changed to The Asylum for the Industrious Blind. In 1876, when the Industrious Blind merged with a society founded by James Gall in 1833 and moved to the present building in Craigmiller Park, "the inauguration was carried out with an amount of military pomp and civic circumstance never known before or since in the world of the blind."

The English were not quite so alert as the Scots in shifting the focus on the blind from the indigent to the industrious, for there is record of the founding of many institutions that carried the word "indigent" in their titles. During the nineteenth century, facilities for the care of the indigent blind continued to increase through private bequest and under voluntary leadership. One of the most notable was the Indigent Blind Visiting Society, founded in 1834 by Lord Shaftesbury and Lord Ebury, with a school for the indigent blind occupying a wing of its premises. New life was injected into the society when Dr. Thomas Rhodes Armitage became a member in 1850 and new workshops for adults were opened in Southwark.

When Dr. Armitage became a member of the Indigent Blind Visiting Society, he established within the organization the "Samaritan Fund," to which he gave £17,000, the income from which was to be used to help blind persons in extreme need. His alert mind soon saw the futility of so much stress being placed on the indigent blind and he determined to try a more positive approach. To accomplish this, he founded in 1868 the British and Foreign Blind Association, which in 1902 became the National Institute for the Blind, now the coördinating organization for many forms of help for the blind in England.

Toward the end of the century, a reaction developed against the voluntary organizations and a demand was made for direct state aid. This was first fomented by a group of blind men, mostly employees in the London workshops, who asserted that the money given and bequeathed by the charitable public for the benefit of the blind was being spent to an undue extent on seeing officials and for management expenses. The group, later organized under the name of the National League for the Blind, further contended "that the problem [of the blind] should be scientifically handled as a whole and not left to the piecemeal action and insufficient resources of the voluntary agencies." ¹ The group became exceedingly aggressive and its propaganda abounded in much hostile criticism of the institutions, or so the officials of these organizations have recorded.

The established voluntary institutions at first fought the plan for government help, maintaining that state aid was not the solution of the problem. At a Conference of Workers for the Blind held in Edinburgh in 1905, it was proposed that the best solution would be to secure contracts for the workshops directly from the government. Substantial orders for baskets and brushes were secured from the Post Office and the War Office, but it was soon discovered that these could not be executed without heavy loss, so the institutions were no better off than before. This forced the committee appointed at Edinburgh to face the situation more realistically, and finally they appealed for state aid. From then on, it was but a matter of framing suitable legislation and in doing this the voluntary institutions and the National League, while differing on details, coöperated in espousing the principle of government assistance for the blind.

In 1914, a motion was proposed in Parliament in the following terms: "That in the opinion of this House, the present voluntary effort in aid of blind people of this country does not adequately meet their necessities, and that the State should make provision whereby capable blind people might be made industrially self-supporting, and the incapable and infirm maintained in a proper and humane manner." ² This led to a recommendation, made in August 1917, that there should be in the Ministry of Health a Central Authority with funds provided by the Exchequer for the general care and supervision of the blind. "This Authority was set up in 1918 and quickly got to grips with its problem." ³

In August 1919, a circular was issued listing the services

for the blind for which grants from the Exchequer would, for the first time, be available. They included workshops, homeworkers' schemes, homes and hostels, home teaching, book production, and support of county associations. For each of these services, a rate of assistance was specified. All of these provisions were incorporated in the Blind Persons Act passed as a Government measure in August 1920.

Some features of this legislation, including later amendments, may be particularly mentioned:

1. Responsibility for the welfare of the blind and also their ascertainment is vested in the Local Authorities throughout the country (that is, the County Councils and County Borough Councils). The Central Authority offers no direct services, but all activities are under the supervision of the Ministry of Health.

2. Many of the services are conducted by the voluntary organizations in continuance of their programs but as agents for the Local Authorities. This includes workshops, homes and hostels, homeworkers' schemes, and home teaching. For these services, the voluntary organizations receive government financial assistance, and the wages of workers in the shops and on homeworkers' schemes are augmented by the government.

3. In recognition of the fact that more than half of the blind are likely to remain unemployed, and that they are not helped by workshops but do require visitation and assistance, responsibility for this service was also placed upon the County Societies. This led to the establishment of the home-teacher scheme.

4. A section of the Blind Persons Act provides for the granting of pensions to the blind at the same rates as Old Age Pensions, except that the blind are eligible for the pensions at the age of fifty rather than seventy as in the case of seeing people. This age was later reduced to forty years.

All in all, this represents an effective way of providing a nation-wide system of welfare for the blind through partnership of central government, local authorities, and voluntary organizations.

All of the provisions of the Blind Persons Act of 1920, and its later amendments, were incorporated in the National Assistance Act of 1948. This was done to relate them to a comprehensive social-security system in which persons with other disabilities are included for the first time: the deaf, the crippled, and others. It is interesting to note that while authorities are *empowered* to provide welfare services for the other handicaps, they are *required* to continue them for the blind.

In 1944, the Disabled Persons (Employment) Act introduced a new feature which requires all firms employing over twenty-five persons to hire a proportion (at present, 3 percent) of disabled workers, including the blind, and to reserve certain occupations entirely for blind persons. This legislation, added to labor shortages, has resulted in the employment in England of more blind persons in open industry than in the sheltered shops or through homeworkers' schemes. The earned wages of all thus employed are augmented by weekly grants from public funds.

While probably no other country in Europe and certainly none in Asia has such a comprehensive program for economic compensation of the blind as England, certain aspects of its services are to be found in many other countries. Some may not be as comprehensive, but one or two (notably that of Canada) are as effective if not better. On the Continent, provision for pensions and some training is universally available for the war-blinded, and gradually the civilian blind are advancing to that status. In 1945, France passed legislation that "envisages" the setting up of rehabilitation centers, but there is little evidence of realization as yet. Most of the European countries have social-security schemes that make some economic provision for the blind. The most certain thing that can be said about economic aid from government sources for blind adults in Europe is that what has been attained has been secured by the efforts of the blind themselves.

In most of the countries of Europe there are now strong associations *of the blind* which have active programs of self-help. In the German Federal Republic, there are several such organizations. The Italian Union for the Blind is a potent group which administers aid in the form of "continuous assistance checks," helps set up blind persons in business, and coöperates with the National Organization of Labor in finding employment for the blind. All of these services are subsidized by government funds. The Association of the Blind in Sweden has its own Sickness and Burial Funds, and the Federation of the Swiss Blind has a scheme for insurance against sickness at greatly reduced rates, and with other organizations assists so that "real need is rare among the blind."

The National Association for the Blind in Spain makes special grants at the time of marriage, maternity, and death, and raises the money for these grants and, at the same time, provides employment for about 9,000 of its estimated 15,000 blind persons, through selling lottery tickets. Anticipating that this form of income might invoke some criticism, the persons answering the questionnaire sent out by the Oxford Conference added: "We are aware that this system of caring for the blind may not commend itself to many of our European colleagues." [4]

13 PARITY—THE GOAL

IN the United States, early efforts to alleviate the lot of the blind differed somewhat from the pattern evolved in the older countries. While an ardent spirit of benevolence abounded in America in the 1830's, there was a definite practicality about the processes and their application. In the field of the blind, projects of practical help were first promoted by seeing people. They have continued to exercise leadership until recently, so that most of the early work in this country may be said to be for the blind rather than by the blind, as was the case abroad.

The work also differs from that in Europe in that it began with greater concern for the industrious blind than for the indigent. The early sighted leaders believed that the blind should work and that the key to open the way to employment was education. But when not enough employers were ready to hire the visually handicapped, there seemed no alternative but economic aid or relief. Later, as the blind became more articulate, they refused to accept either education or relief as final answers. Today a growing leadership of competent blind persons is seeking new ways. Granting that schooling is the right of all, and relief a necessity for the indigent, the industrious blind are asking for a handicap allowance that will give them economic parity and maintain their self-respect.

Financial aid for the indigent blind, based largely on the concept of relief for the poor established through legislation in 1601 under Queen Elizabeth I, did not arise in this country until 1866, when New York City first allocated public funds to assist blind persons. This late development was not due to any lack of humane interest in the welfare of those with restricted vision, but rather was the result of the optimistic hope of the early pioneers that, with adequate training, blind persons could and should be contributing members of society. Samuel Gridley Howe's early observations convinced him that in Europe there was too much charity and segregation and not enough compulsion to work and integration into the community.

In his first report in 1832, Dr. Howe wrote:

> Instead of condemning the poor blind man to stand at the corner of the street and ask for charity . . . you may give to him the means of becoming an enlightened, happy, and useful member of society; you may give him and his fellow blind the means of earning their own livelihood or at least doing much toward it . . . The object is an economical one to the community. It is to take from society so many "dead weights" that it is proposed to educate the blind and enable them to earn their own livelihood; and society ought to consider any capital so invested as a sinking fund for the redemption of its charitable debts; as a provision for preventing the blind from becoming taxes to the community.[1]

Dr. Howe reavowed this conviction throughout his life, but there are some indications that at times his faith faltered. Within ten years of the opening of Perkins Institution, he encountered difficulty in finding employment for those who had completed their schooling. It is evident that he did not attribute this difficulty to inability or lack of desire to work on the part of the blind people, but rather to the reluctance of the seeing to hire them. To counteract this reluctance and to educate the seeing employers, Dr. Howe opened in Boston in 1840 the first workshop for the blind in this country. Its primary purpose was not to provide employment but to demonstrate the capabilities of the trained blind.

At first, the men lived in the school, but in 1880 they were required to live outside in rooms of their own, partly because of their bad example to the younger pupils, but chiefly as a first step in their fuller integration into the community. Perkins continued to operate the workshop, primarily for the making and remaking of mattresses, until 1952, when it was closed partly because of difficulty in securing work to do (as

cotton and foam rubber are replacing the hair mattress) and
partly because of the equal difficulty of getting blind persons
to work in the shop now that open employment and direct
financial aid are more easily secured. In a way it had fulfilled
its purpose.

The workshop idea as a medium of employment and a
means of economic compensation for visual impairment has
grown in America. The shops here, however, differ from
those in Europe in that they are in no way associated with
the schools. In fact, few of the employees are former students
of schools for the blind but are people who have lost their
sight later in life. Many of the shops are now used for the
retraining of the newly blinded, and their objective is to
return to open industry as many workers as possible. Originally, the shops were truly "sheltered"; that is, they provided
a place for the blind person of limited ability to be sheltered
from the speed and stresses of modern industry. While the
work produced in the shops is expected to be of commercial
quality, the quantity is not supposed to meet commercial
standards, especially in shops where only the marginal workers are retained. For that reason, "sheltered" workshops for
the blind have to be subsidized and in some shops it costs a
dollar to pay a dollar to the worker.

Most of the shops in this country are owned and operated
by private organizations and are supported by voluntary contributions. A few shops, particularly the older ones, provide
residences for the workers: the Pennsylvania Home for Blind
Women (1868) and the Pennsylvania Working Home for
Blind Men (1874), both in Philadelphia; the Industrial
Home for the Adult Blind (now known as the Training Center for the Adult Blind) in Oakland, California (1885); the
Industrial Home for the Blind in Brooklyn (1897); the
Clovernook Home for Blind Women in Cincinnati (1903);
and the Michigan Employment Institution for the Blind in
Saginaw (1905). Other shops are but a small part of the total
programs of supporting organizations. The Lighthouse of
New York, for example, provides many forms of personal
service, as well as entertainment, education, and recreation.

It also administers for the state the assistance program within the city. Founded in 1905 by Mrs. Winifred Holt Mather, it has counterparts in many parts of the world.

It is characteristic of the approach to blindness in this country that the first efforts to help the visually handicapped on the national level were based on educational programs rather than on those concerned with social welfare. The American Association of Instructors of the Blind, whose leadership and membership has from the beginning been largely composed of seeing people, was established in 1853. In its activities, the A. A. I. B. has strictly adhered to the field of education. In England, the Association of Teachers of the Blind was not organized until 1912, whereas the National League of the Blind, which fostered the Blind Persons Act of 1920, was founded by blind persons in 1893.

Perhaps equally characteristic of the American approach is the fact that the first organization of blind people in the United States was not founded until 1895. An early name, American Blind People's Higher Education and General Improvement Association, implied that the goals of larger opportunity that they were seeking were to come through more education. After a battle with the educators on the multiplicity of types, the group with the long name reorganized and became in 1905 the present American Association of Workers for the Blind.

"This Association," wrote Dr. French,

constituted itself the merciless, but not altogether undiscerning, critic of all that *was* representative of the older institutionalism. Its work has been to force uniformity of type on a reluctant educational system, to foster agencies for the employment of the blind under conditions permitting home life and the normal contacts, and either to re-form and modernize or dispense with the specialized institutions . . . It is perhaps well that the A. A. W. B. should continue to be the "Party of the Opposition." [2]

As in England, there came a time in the United States when it was felt that an agency was needed to coördinate all types of voluntary work for the blind. First proposed in 1909, the idea crystallized in 1921, when representatives of the American Association of Instructors of the Blind and the American Association of Workers for the Blind united in bringing into being the American Foundation for the Blind. This fulfilled many of the functions of the National Institute for the Blind in England. Like its older brother, the younger organization was led through its formative years by a blind executive, Robert B. Irwin, who became associated with the Foundation in 1923 and continued there until his retirement in 1949. During this period, the Foundation developed manifold activities and became a potent factor in all phases of work for the blind through the active leadership of Dr. Irwin and the generous patronage of Major M. C. Migel.

Robert B. Irwin, born in Rockford, Iowa, on June 3, 1883, was brought up in the pioneer community of Vaughn on Puget Sound in the State of Washington. He differed from his counterpart in England, Dr. Armitage, in that he lost his sight early, at the age of five; but Irwin had much of the same zeal and was always ready for a crusade if it would benefit the sightless. At the age of seven, young Irwin was sent to the state school for the blind. In after years, he used to say, with a twinkle in his voice which did not completely cover the bitterness that he felt, that he had been educated at the "School for Defective Youth," as the institution which included the blind was then called. He, however, was graduated in 1901 and proceeded to the University of Washington, earning his B. A. degree in 1906, followed by the attainment of a Master of Arts degree in the field of education at Harvard in 1907.

Irwin's interests as head of the foundation soon reached beyond the blind of this country. Under his leadership, the Foundation sponsored the World Conference of Work for the Blind held in New York City in April 1931. This gathering did much to renew ties in this special field of humane interest which had been severed by World War I. Later, Dr. Irwin was largely instrumental in creating the American Foundation for Overseas Blind which, on February 5, 1946, took over the obligations and program of the American Braille

Press for War and Civilian Blind which had been founded in 1915 by American interests in France at the time of World War I. On March 15, 1952, the activities and assets of the Association for the Chinese Blind were merged with the program of the Overseas Blind.

After World War II, Irwin was chairman of an organizing committee appointed by the American Foundation for Overseas Blind and the National Institute of the Blind of England to convene a conference of workers with the adult blind. This was held at Merton College, Oxford University, in the summer of 1949, with nineteen nations represented. At this gathering, a program of minimum standards for work with the blind was set up. This was presented to and later adopted by the United Nations.

It was not until the twentieth century that this country really came to grips with blindness as a governmental responsibility and the officials were spurred into this by the voluntary workers. In 1903, a group of Boston people concerned over the difficulties encountered by the blind after school age formed an organization whose name well describes its purpose: The Massachusetts Association for Promoting the Interests of the Adult Blind. While its primary objective was to render assistance to the adult blind through home teaching and provision for personal services, it soon began to agitate for a state program for the blind. This led to the establishment in 1906 of the Massachusetts Commission for the Blind, the first permanent state agency for the adult blind in this country.

In 1893, Connecticut formed a Board of Education for the Blind in accord with the earlier emphasis on education as the medium of help, while in the same year that the Massachusetts Commission was authorized the State of Illinois enacted legislation known as the "blind pension bill" which made possible direct financial aid to the blind as a measure of social welfare. The Illinois program was organized under the Department of Welfare, whereas the Massachusetts Commission was changed in 1920 from an independent agency to a division of the State Department of Education. In the first third of the century, twenty-six states set up state-supported agencies for the blind following one or the other of the patterns, either under Welfare or under Education.

It took the social sweep of the New Deal to bring to the blind any measure of national recognition and assistance. The only federal aid to the blind prior to that time was the allocation in 1879 of $10,000 annually to provide textbooks and appliances for schools for the blind. In 1931, legislation was passed authorizing funds to provide reading matter for the adult blind. The blind shared in the benefits of WPA and other relief enterprises but not to any greater extent than the seeing. Projects were set up giving indirect benefits such as the making of maps and models for schools for the blind, while others were created for the sole purpose of giving the sightless a chance to work and receive direct compensation. In order to prevent the repetition of social conditions revealed during the depression of the 1930's, the Social Security Act of 1935 was enacted.

When the Social Security Act was being formulated, organized forces of workers for the blind were determined to see that those without sight should receive their full share. Leaders in this field insisted that the blind should not be included in the general category of the needy but that their peculiar status should be separately recognized. This led to the introduction of Title X within the Social Security Act, which gave as its purpose "to furnish financial assistance to needy individuals who are blind." This followed the pattern of Title I, providing old-age assistance, rather than that of Title V, covering assistance for crippled children, including medical care.

An amendment to broaden the scope of Title X so that states could be reimbursed for expenses of "locating blind persons, providing eye diagnoses, and for the training and employment of the adult blind" was stricken out at a joint congressional conference largely on the emotional attitude that the blind should not be expected to work but that provision should be made to help them through direct financial assistance. Based on this philosophy, Title X in its original form was limited to 50 percent reimbursement to states for money spent in aid of the needy blind, up to a maximum of $30 a month to any one individual. This formula has been raised through subsequent amendments. In 1952, provision was made for reimbursement to the states for four-fifths of the first $25 and one-half of the remainder of a grant up to a total of $55. For assistance beyond this maximum, payment may be made through state funds.

Under the terms of the Social Security Act, aid to the blind was to be administered by state agencies conforming to federal requirements. In most cases, this work fell to the State Departments of Welfare, although in four states, Massachusetts, New Jersey, Missouri, and Delaware, aid is fully administered by state agencies for the blind, and in North Carolina, Virginia, and Washington, state divisions of the blind supervise the grants paid by the Departments of Welfare. Under the stimulus of federal participation, the number of states providing aid for the needy blind increased from twenty-six in 1935 to forty-eight in 1953, when Nevada met requirements and completed the roster of states.

Workers for the blind generally felt that the intended benefits under Social Security were not fully attained. In fact, to many it seemed like retrogression to the old policy of rewarding the indigent and penalizing the industrious. For under this plan, one blind person might do some work and make, possibly, $25 a month, while his blind neighbor might sit in his rocking chair and at the end of the month each would have the same amount of money, since Title X, as first enacted, required that all sums earned or received be deducted from the monthly allotment. This form of assistance removed the incentive to work unless it was possible to earn more than the assistance grant. Certainly this provision did little to reward diligent workers or to encourage thrift.

In 1950, an effort was made to correct this situation, for in that year Title X was amended so that in allocating assistance, earnings up to $50 a month were made exempt. Through this amendment the industrious blind person of limited ability at least became somewhat better off than his indigent neighbor. But there is still an inherent danger that the blind person might stop work when he has earned $49.50 in order to get his assistance rather than press on to attain possible maximum earnings. Increasing the earned exemption, however, is not the way to encourage full employment; in fact, it only cuts down the incentive to go off relief.

Some states have endeavored to remedy the inequities of public-assistance policy by providing a special system of grants which encourage earnings on the grounds that it is better to give more financial assistance to a man who has the potential of becoming self-supporting through this help than to one who will make no effort to earn his own way. California has provision to supplement assistance under Title X through additional aid from state funds. Massachusetts has the same power, which was exercised largely in promoting self-help until 1940, when by legislation $40 a month was fixed as minimum assistance. Pennsylvania in 1935 authorized the supplementation of income for all of the blind in the state. This was amended in 1952 so that every blind person is assured of an annual income of $1,716.

Under this supplementary legislative permission, Pennsylvania leads all states in the number of individuals aided and Massachusetts tops all in the size of the average grant. In December 1954, Pennsylvania aided, with an average grant of $50.88, 16,354 of its 19,947 (figure as of July 1, 1952) blind citizens, but 7,530 were assisted without federal participation. Massachusetts' average grant at the end of 1954 was $92.12, but it assisted only 1,782 of its 7,864 blind. Until recently, California usually led in both categories, but in December 1954, it was second in the number of participants: 12,396 of its 19,363 blind, and only 410 were aided without federal contribution. It was third in the average payment, $84.82, being exceeded by New York with its average grant of $86.11 made to 4,380 of its 25,501 blind. The lowest average state grant was made by Mississippi, $34.27, paid to 3,396 of its 6,432 blind persons.

It is interesting to note the differences in the ratio of blind persons helped in the several states. In addition to those cited above there are other wide variations. New Jersey with 8,522 blind citizens aided only 861 under Title X and Connecticut assisted 310 of its 3,197 blind. Illinois with 15,250 blind persons assisted 3,601, while Georgia with 9,174 helped practically the same number, 3,303 of its blind persons. These variations are not to be attributed to parsimony or generosity but to the effectiveness of promoting measures of self-help.

Further study of aid to the needy blind under the provisions of Title X of the Social Security Act shows that, including state supplementation, an average grant of $56.37 was paid in December 1954 to 102,445 blind persons at a total cost of $5,774,614. To grasp the full significance of this aid, it is necessary to give the cost for a full year. "To furnish financial assistance to needy individuals who are blind," the objective set forth when the Social Security Act was enacted in 1935, plus certain medical care, cost, in the year 1954, $68,350,228!

But even more significant than the money spent is the large number of persons, over 100,000, who, by virtue of receiving these grants, are classified as needy or at least as not earning over $50 a month. With approximately 300,000 blind persons in this country, one-third are now, according to the statistics of Social Security, within the category of the indigent. Even though over $60,000,000 a year is spent under Title X of the Social Security Act, it does not give to the blind what they want above all else: the right and opportunity to work. "Idleness, not blindness," Helen Keller has often said, "is what the blind find hardest to bear."

Workers for the blind and the blind themselves are not content with this legislation and are continuing their efforts for a sounder program of national financial support and for the strengthening of the broad programs of the more progressive states. Some of this desired help came in 1943 when the Congress enacted legislation enlarging the scope of the Vocational Rehabilitation Act of 1920. Passed during World War II, this legislation was intended to make provision for the rehabilitation of both civilians and those disabled in the armed services. In a special message to Congress, President

Roosevelt made that request, and the Barden-LaFollette Bill was originally so framed. But the ink had hardly dried on the printed document when the veterans' lobby deleted the provisions for the war disabled. These were incorporated in the Clark-Walsh Bill, which was quickly enacted as Public Law 16, March 24, 1943, under which aid to the war disabled, including the blind, is administered by the Veterans Administration. Provision for civilian rehabilitation was enacted as Public Law 113 on September 8, 1943.

The great forward step under Public Law 113 was that it provided federal funds on a fifty-fifty basis for "any services necessary to render a disabled individual fit to engage in a remunerative occupation." Under the old legislation, rehabilitation workers used to say that they had to work around a disability, while under the new law they could work through a disability. For example, formerly, if a man had lost a leg, the workers had to find a job that could be done by a one-legged person; now, they have funds to provide an artificial limb and to make the man a two-legged worker.

Likewise, formerly, if a person was visually handicapped because of cataract, all that many states could or would do was to give him a pension and retire him from active work. Funds are now available to have the cataracts removed and the man restored to normal activity. This legislation reimburses the states for one-half of all that they expend in giving medical examinations to employable visually handicapped persons and for providing medical and surgical care, hospitalization, and prosthetic devices for those who pass a means test, that is, who are unable to pay. The same reimbursement is given for rehabilitation training with provision for maintenance and transportation during instruction.

In order to promote, above all else, the employment of blind persons, federal funds were made available for the full costs of counseling and placement services. The law also provides for that part of the program pertaining to the blind to be administered by existing state agencies, with the Federal Government reimbursing the states for all expenses incurred in the administration of the program. Since the enactment of this law, all states have accepted participation, although many still operate under partial programs, owing to the insufficiency of state appropriations.

For the administration of the program under Public Law 113 at the federal level, the Office of Vocational Rehabilitation with a Section for the Blind was set up in the Social Security Board, which in 1953 became the Department of Health, Education, and Welfare. One of the first projects of the Section for the Blind was to hold courses for the training of counselors and placement officers so that the expanding state programs would have qualified personnel. They have also established standards and listed jobs suitable for blind workers.

The "rehab" workers claim that the expenditure for rehabilitation has a high return in wages earned and taxes paid, estimating that for each dollar spent, ten dollars comes back as taxes paid on earnings. These figures are hard to sustain and the exact number of blind persons permanently rehabilitated is difficult to ascertain because there is inadequate provision for follow-up on placements, and the total number reported may well include a considerable number of "repeats." Dr. Howard Rusk, the eminent authority on rehabilitation, warns, however, that "if we do not use the disabled, by 1980 every able-bodied worker will be carrying one physically handicapped, one chronically ill, and one worker beyond sixty-five, on his back."

What the blind are now seeking, with some support from sighted workers, is economic parity with the seeing. This, the visually handicapped feel, is essential as a first step toward social integration. It is generally accepted that there are costs of living inherent in blindness which exceed similar expenses for the seeing. For that reason, the blind claim, there should be specific compensation for the loss of sight. This compensation, however, should not be considered as relief associated with indigency or looked upon as a pension which implies retirement from the active world, but rather as a handicap allowance that gives to blind people a fairer chance to compete with the seeing. Some of the legislation enacted during this century has had that objective in view.

The Randolph-Sheppard Act of 1936 authorized the opening of vending stands in public buildings for the sale of newspapers, periodicals, confections, and tobacco products for operation solely by blind persons. The Wagner-O'Day Act of 1938 requires departments of the Federal Government to buy as needed, at a fair market price, from workshops for the blind such articles as brooms, mops, and other products of blind labor. This resulted in a great boom for the shops, especially during the war, when it was reported that the workshops made and hemmed almost fifty million pillowcases and nearly as many sheets. Some of the states are setting up little Wagner-O'Day Acts to capture some of this business on the state level.

Prior to that legislation, however, Massachusetts and Indiana had laws requiring state institutions to purchase products made by the blind. Massachusetts now requires all publicly owned pianos to be serviced by blind tuners. In 1940, an amendment was attached to the Income Tax Law that permitted the deduction of $500 for special expenses incurred as a result of blindness. This has since been advanced to $600. On nearly all railroad and bus lines, a blind person and guide may travel on trains and busses paying only one fare. Recently the State of Washington authorized the issuing of free licenses for hunting and fishing to all veterans and blind persons, and then added reflectively that, when issued to blind persons, the license shall be "limited to fishing only."

Today many people genuinely interested in the sightless are not too happy about all of the special legislation enacted in the first half of this century. Too much of it has been based on emotion and not enough on the competence of modern social practice. There is also the growing fear that increasing benefits attained in this way are making the blind a segregated class and are halting progress toward the ideal: integration with the seeing. Integration works two ways, for it must not be overlooked that the sighted have a stake in an adequate and comprehensive plan of care for the blind. Enlightened leaders, both sighted and blind, are now seeking a way to off-set the dire consequences of impairment of vision that will cover not only those now without sight but also those who day by day will lose their sight.

A plan that would seem to accomplish this aim was advo-cated by the late Robert B. Irwin, who proposed that in addi-tion to Title X there should be in the Social Security Act a plan for insurance against blindness modeled after Old Age and Survivors Insurance with adaptations for the special needs of the blind. An average of two cents a day for each wage earner, one cent paid by the employee and the other by the employer, would yield, Dr. Irwin claimed, to each per-son covered by Social Security the assurance of $40 a month on becoming blind. Quite apart from the validity of these figures, which are now out of date, the principle is one to which consideration should be given. This would not be legislation for the blind as a separate class, but for all people, who in this way could prepare for the possibility of blindness as the prudent arrange for financial security in old age and for insurance payable upon death. It would not be a pension or relief given out of compassion but an income earned, carrying with it the self-respect of the individual and the rec-ognition of society's responsibility for the prevalence of blind-ness.

As this plan would provide only for those coming under Social Security, there would have to be provision for those not covered, and for those who are born blind or who lose their sight before reaching working years. Dr. Irwin had an answer for that. His plan called for setting up a special fund for these groups and for what the insurance actuaries call "ac-crued liabilities." For the accumulation and maintenance of this fund, he proposed a tax on electric light bulbs, receipts from which would be definitely designated for assistance to the blind under the Insurance Against Blindness plan. While Dr. Irwin's suggestion has a certain poetic justice, it is not an entirely new idea.

In 1882, Edward Everett Hale, speaking at Perkins Institution, pleaded that the blind might have "equality before the law" which is assured in the Constitution. This, he stated, the blind do not have when money they are required to pay in taxes is used to provide "these long ribbons of lights—extending North, South, East, and West—like a cobweb laid over the whole city lighted up every night as the lamplighter makes his rounds." [3]

14 THE TOLL OF WAR

As one reviews the social and economic schemes provided for the sightless one is soon aware that an objective of the leaders of the civilian blind is to bring their benefits up to the level attained by the war blinded. For it is true that in all countries those who lost their sight in war service hold a preferred position. Although as time passes the glory accorded to the man who gave his sight for his country fades and he becomes, in the peace time community, just another man who cannot see, he still has continued preferment through higher financial aid, job security, and hospital care. High sympathy for the war blind is easy to understand and no one would deny them all that society can do to compensate for their loss. But the civilian blind have a point when they claim that loss of sight through the hazards of peace is equally the responsibility of society.

Veteran preferment, however, in all categories of disablement, has a long history and in recent years it has been built up into a potent political force. When this began is hard to say. Perhaps the great Byzantine general, Belisarius, one of the legendary figures of the sixth century, may have been the first blinded warrior. His loss of sight, however, was not incurred in conflict, for legend has it that the Emperor Justinian ordered him blinded, since he outshone the emperor in popularity because of his victories in battle. Despite his fame as a soldier, he ended his days begging on the streets of Constantinople and his call "A penny for Belisarius the General" continued a saying long after his time. Or possibly General Johann Zizka may be preferred as the first blind veteran. A great Bohemian patriot, he was more feared after he lost his sight than before. Without sight he led his troops in a battle at Kamnitz in 1422 that established the freedom of his country. He died, however, not in service but from the plague, on October 11, 1425, a blind veteran truly honored and highly esteemed.

Special provision for warriors who lost their sight may be said to have begun when Louis IX is reputed to have provided asylum for three hundred blind crusaders in Paris in 1254, endowed them with privileges, and granted freedom from taxation. Germany, in 1813, when trachoma was taking its toll of sight among the troops returned from the Napoleonic wars in Egypt, set up compensation for blindness, and England, in 1818, opened a special hospital for men with impaired vision and provided financial assistance to those who had lost their sight from what was then called military ophthalmia.

In this country, provision for maimed soldiers was first decreed by the Pilgrim Courts in 1636 when it was ruled that they should be cared for for life. Similar, but not as generous, acts were passed by the Virginia Assembly in 1664 and by the Maryland Militia in 1678. In the Massachusetts Bay Colony compensation for injured soldiers was determined in Town Meeting. The first National Disability Law was passed by the Continental Congress on August 26, 1776. This called for a maximum of half pay for those so disabled as not to be able to earn a living. Payment of this compensation fell upon the states, but the Congress made grants of land up to 1000 acres, according to length of service and of rank. At the time of the War of 1812 the Navy, independent of the Army, set up its own pension system which was financed by money received from prizes of war. Payments to sailors from this source were more regular than those made to soldiers from government funds.

Blindness as a specific cause for compensation in the pension system was first recognized by legislation enacted on July 4, 1864. For the loss of both eyes a veteran was entitled to $25 a month. This sum was increased gradually up to and following the Spanish-American War, but the number of pensioners rose in greater proportion owing largely to the salesmanship of claim agents. It was not, however, until World War I that war blindness became recognized as a disability requiring specially organized programs of training, rehabilitation, and placement, as well as aftercare often lasting through life. For as Eugène Brieux, the distinguished member of the Academy of Sciences who took charge of retraining the French blind, wrote, "For some wounded our responsibility is over when their wounds healed, but with the blind it only begins. . . . They need to be prepared for their new life."

The impact of blindness as a serious war casualty was of course first felt in France. The medical departments of the allied armies were prepared to deal with the surgical aspects of eye damage but were without experience or facilities to provide the retraining and aftercare which, as M. Brieux pointed out, made the blind different from the other wounded. France turned immediately to the oldest foundation for the sightless, the Hospice des Quinze-Vingts, which at the time maintained an eye clinic. This had been considerably expanded in 1913. On August 24, 1914 this historic home for the blind was converted into a military hospital and its 300 beds were occupied by eye and face casualties. When all possible medical care had been given, the healed were discharged and the blind remained. What should be done with them? Were they to remain for the rest of their lives with all the privileges made available for three hundred blind men by Louis IX in 1254?

Something new and drastic had to be done and France was fortunate in having able men like J. Brisac, director of the Department of Public Aid and Hygiene in the Ministry of the Interior, and Eugène Brieux ready to undertake the task. An Annex to the Hospice was set up, and an organization called "Friends of Blinded Soldiers" was established under the leadership of René Vallery-Radot. The society was organized on March 29, 1915 and on the same day a center for forty soldiers was opened in a house ten years abandoned on the Rue Reuilly. The property was situated in a park of over twelve acres and as the air in Reuilly is reputed to be pure it was considered a suitable refuge for blinded soldiers. Despite the handicap of a dilapidated building a program was developed and to the limit of its capacity a plan of convalescence, retraining, and shop work was undertaken.

When the École de Reuilly was opened it was thought that the war would soon be over and that the available space would be adequate. But as the war continued and when the Army Medical Department ordered that all blinded soldiers be sent to Reuilly it was soon evident that more room was required. As the authorities studied the situation it was learned that the vast majority of cases were peasants or agricultural workers whose main desire was to go home. It was therefore decided to open simpler training centers in the provinces. Seventeen were conducted during the war and through them passed most of the 2800 blinded servicemen of France. Several other efforts to help the war blinded were undertaken in France by other national groups. Volunteers from the United States went over to serve in the hospitals, and special centers were set up. Outstanding was the opening of The Lighthouse by Miss Winifred Holt, later Mrs. Rufus Mather, which still carries on, and the American Braille Press, which continued to produce reading matter until its merger with the American Foundation of Overseas Blind in 1946.

Neither available information nor space will permit a full account of how all the warring nations undertook to prepare their blinded service men and women for life in the darkened world in which they must thereafter live. But a few will be described. Belgium, as an example of the smaller nations, set up its program for the retraining of blinded soldiers within the army. The men were continued in uniform, discipline was maintained, and training was required. The problem proved not too difficult, for fewer than one hundred men were involved. Germany, with the largest number of blinded soldiers, had about 7000 to retain. Unique features of the reëducation program were the training of guide dogs, now widely used in many countries, legislation requiring industry to employ a quota of disabled persons, and the development of a special school at Marburg to prepare the qualified for the university. Compensation by the government was based on the cost of living in the region where the veteran lived. Italy had nearly 3000 eye casualties. These were concentrated in three hospitals at Milan, Florence, and Rome. On completion of medical care the men were distributed among six reëducation institutes, some of which were existing schools for the blind. An organization was formed to help with aftercare and some of the workshops opened have been continued for blinded veterans. In the school at Rome, directed by Professor Romagnoli, a distinguished blind teacher, a course in "orientation" was obligatory for all.

England's program for its war blinded, of whom there were nearly 3000, was not a government undertaking but was promoted and supported by a voluntary agency which continues to the present time, under the name of St. Dunstan's. A large factor in the success of the program was the fortunate choice of its founder, Arthur Pearson, a prominent journalist who had to leave Fleet Street because of failing sight. He had become associated with the National Institute for the Blind when the war came on and wounded soldiers began to reach London. "The main idea that animated me," wrote Sir Arthur (for he was later knighted for his work at St. Dunstan's), "in establishing this Hostel for the blinded soldiers was that the sightless men, after being discharged from the hospital, might come into a little world where the things which a blind person cannot do were forgotten and where everyone was concerned with what blind people can do." [1]

"I wanted delightful surroundings," asserted Pearson, and he found them in the magnificent estate of the American banker, Otto Kahn, situated in the Inner Circle of Regent's Park, London. The mansion with fifteen acres of gardens and grounds, larger than any in London save Buckingham

Palace, was maintained by Mr. Kahn throughout the war. Pearson began his work with sixteen blinded servicemen on March 26, 1915. As the work grew, other buildings were acquired and later convalescent homes were opened at Brighton and St. Leonards-on-Sea. "With practically no exception," wrote Sir Arthur, in his book *Victory Over Blindness*, "all the soldiers and sailors of the British Imperial Forces blinded in the war came under my care to learn how to be blind." [2]

While the impelling force in the retraining of the blind at St. Dunstan's was the inspiring personality of its leader, there were certain principles that made the program successful. Men were not admitted to St. Dunstan's until the completion of medical care. It was arranged, however, for all blinded servicemen upon reaching England to be centered at nearby St. Mark's Hospital, Chelsea (the 2nd London General Hospital) where they were immediately visited by workers from St. Dunstan's. First contacts aimed at teaching men how to be blind: how to eat, how to shave, to light a cigarette, and perform other daily tasks. When moved to St. Dunstan's they were given opportunity to train for the days ahead. In addition to learning braille and the traditional skills for the blind, new fields were explored with success.

So impresed were government authorities with this training program that St. Dunstan's was allowed to administer and make payment of pensions to men while under training. Its leaders have continued to advocate enlargement of compensation for loss of sight among veterans. Financial aid available under government regulations is granted, not at a uniform rate according to physical loss sustained, but according to the rank of the men while in service. These grants are frequently supplemented by St. Dunstan's in order to attain their objective of enabling each man to make the most of his training or to carry on as nearly as possible under the same economic conditions as prevailed before he entered service. To assist further their men St. Dunstan's set up an extensive aftercare program which has grown into one of the most valuable features of England's plan for its war blinded. At the time of the armistice of World War I, 1,300 men were under the care of St. Dunstan's and over the years 1,500 more veterans of that war were admitted. And in 1954, 1,450 were still being served, of whom 63 percent were reported to be still working, most of them probably in home industries rather than in industrial employment.

The United States was not as fortunate in its program in World War I, but it had only one-tenth as many blinded, slightly under 300, compared with nearly 3,000 in England. In addition much of the initial work was done in France by Americans who went over for that purpose and a few men were cared for at St. Dunstan's. It took some time to get any program under way in this country. First, the extent of the need had not been anticipated, and second, it was thought that provision for all war casualties would be covered by the War Risk Insurance Act of 1914 as amended in 1917. The purpose of this legislation was to provide, through insurance, indemnities as a substitute for pensions, which, Harry Best wrote, was "a novel feature in American military effort." [3]

Under the Bureau of War Risk Insurance there was established a Division of Military and Naval Insurance which had authority to grant disability allowances to officers and enlisted men who suffered injury or contracted disease "in the line of duty," and "when employed in active service under the War Department or Navy Department." This provided for blindness or the loss of sight in both eyes: specifically, the sum of $100 a month is granted to be payable through life, with no other compensation. For partial disability the allowance is based on the loss of earning power (with no allowance if this loss is less than 10 percent) , as determined by average impairments in civil occupations, and not on individual impairments, so that there may be no reduction for individual success in overcoming handicaps.[4]

As is well known, this "novel feature in American military effort" of indemnity through insurance as a substitute for pensions from public funds was soon thrown aside and legislation for ever-increasing compensation went marching on.

In the meantime the military authorities were confronted with blinded casualties and a program had to be devised. At a conference called by the Committee on Ophthalmology of the Council of National Defense in October 1917, representatives of the Surgeon General and educators of and workers for the blind, a plan based on three stages of curative and restorative treatment was approved. The first stage was to be carried on in hospitals immediately after disablement, where, in addition to all medical and surgical care, occupational therapy was planned and recreational facilities were provided. After all possible medical care was completed, patients found to be permanently blind were to be transferred to the second stage to be conducted at a special center where vocational training was to be undertaken and plans were to be made for transition back to civilian life. To carry out the third stage, when the blinded men were discharged from the Army and returned to their home communities, the Federal Board for Vocational Education was created in 1918. Its purpose was to develop, through federal aid to states, programs of vocational training that would enable a person "to carry on a gainful occupation, to resume his former occupation, or to enter some other occupation."

The heart of the whole plan was, of course, in the second stage. For a training center, Mrs. T. Harrison Garrett offered, in November 1917, her estate at Guilford, near Baltimore, known as Evergreen. Opened in April 1918 as U. S. Army General Hospital No. 7, this venture never seemed to find itself or to be able to fulfill adequately its intended purpose. There were a number of reasons. It never had the strong leadership that made St. Dunstan's so effective. The projects of training were not realistic. For example, it was proposed that an ideal occupation for blinded veterans might be found in chain stores, whereupon men were trained for that work without any attempt to explore the possibilities of placement. It is said that one staff worker, to lift the morale of the men and to make the seeing world think that the trainees were not blind, had them carry books under their arms when they went to Baltimore. To supplement the program of the Army and to bring to the men the flexibility found in voluntary organizations, the American Red Cross opened a center on an estate adjoining Evergreen. Here provision was made for friendly recreation, and families of the men were invited to visit to become acquainted with the ways of the blind. Through local chapters the Red Cross did much to facilitate the transfer back to home communities. It also acted as an intermediary between the military training school and the Federal Board for Vocational Education.

Because of low morale among those enrolled in the hospital, the reluctance of others to forego pensions surpassing army pay, and problems of administration, the center was transferred from the Army to the control of the Federal Board of Vocational Rehabilitation and the Red Cross Institute for the Blinded on January 1, 1919. Under the direction of the latter, physical changes were made and equipment added at a cost of $1,000,000. More extensive courses for the men were set up and studies of industrial possibilities for the blind were made. Perhaps one of the best contributions of the project were the monographs on the war blinded in this and other countries prepared and published by the Institute. On January 1, 1922 the Veterans Administration took control and operated the center under the same program until it was finally closed on May 1, 1925.

During World War I, discharged soldiers and sailors had to deal with three different government agencies: the medical department for professional care, the Bureau of Pensions for financial aid, and the Board for Vocational Education for occupational training. This led to so much confusion that in 1921 the President appointed a committee to make an inquiry into the administration of all laws providing for the care of disabled servicemen. This resulted in the creation of the Veterans Bureau as an independent agency in 1921. In 1930, by executive order, all facilities for veterans were consolidated under the Veterans Administration. From that time until World War II all provision for blinded veterans was in the hands of the Veterans Administration.

The chief form of help has been financial aid through

pensions as established by law for varying degrees of loss of sight. A smaller number of men have been given domiciliary care in homes for veterans. Although there were only about 300 blind casualties in World War I, that number has increased through the years, partly because of the normal advance in blindness in old age and partly because of the VA practice of extending assistance for nonservice-incurred disabilities. General Frank T. Hines, for many years head of the Veterans Administration, reported on September 13, 1944 that "there are a total of 3648 veterans on the compensation and pension rolls who are totally blind or have not more than 20/200 vision in the better eye." A study made in 1946 indicated that there were in Veterans Administration hospitals and homes 337 blinded men, of whom 8 were veterans of World War II, 307 of World War I, and 14 of the Spanish-American War. The others lost their sight from nonservice-connected causes.

When World War II broke out, England had the advantage over other countries in that St. Dunstan's was fully operating. Its effective program of aftercare was functioning and through it over 2000 of the blinded of World War I were still being served. Between the wars the beautiful convalescent home built on the hillside overlooking the Atlantic near Brighton was available for any St. Dunstaners feeling the need of rest and recreation, while in the neighboring village of Ovingdean there was a vacation nursery for the children of blinded veterans. The home industries with sales outlets in London were thriving. St. Dunstan's was ready with necessary facilities and personnel.

St. Dunstan's was fortunate also in its leadership. Sir Arthur Pearson had been succeeded in 1921 by Lt. Col. Sir Ian Fraser, a product of St. Dunstan's. When only eighteen Fraser was blinded in the Battle of the Somme. After completing training at St. Dunstan's he qualified as a barrister and entered Parliament in his early twenties. For many years Sir Ian was a governor of the British Broadcasting Corporation and now (1955) is president of the British Legion. Holding these positions, Sir Ian has been able to press the cause of the disabled on British public opinion and to obtain many reforms for the blind through acts of Parliament. Immediately upon the outbreak of war in 1939, Sir Ian set the wheels in motion for the reception of blinded casualties. The beautiful home in Brighton and the London centers soon had to be abandoned because of air raids. A new center was opened in a large resort hotel in the village of Church Stretton in Shropshire south of Shrewsbury. Here over 1000 men and women received training during the war, of whom 300 regained useful vision. In 1954, 1100 veterans of World War II were under the care of St. Dunstan's, and it was reported that only 10 percent were not doing remunerative work.

To extend its facilities and to provide more immediate service, outposts were set up by St. Dunstan's during World War II in South Africa, Egypt, and Italy, and a center was opened at Dehra Dun in India under the leadership of Sir Clutha MacKenzie, a New Zealander who lost his sight in World War I and was retrained at St. Dunstan's. Another St. Dunstaner of distinction, Lt. Col. E. O. Baker, M.C., O.B.E., managing director of the Canadian Institute for the Blind, undertook to retrain the war blinded of the Dominion in a program carried on at the Canadian National Institute in Toronto. Here at the close of the war 158 men and women had received training, 110 from the European and Middle East battlefields and 40 from the Hong Kong prisoner of war group. Among the last a new form of loss of sight, from malnutrition, augmented the total war casualties.

England faced another cause of war blindness that called for special treatment. This was among civilians who were the victims of air raids. Two hundred forty-seven persons suffered loss of sight in this way. To care for them the National Institute for the Blind opened three centers called "Homes of Recovery." They were not hospitals or training centers but rather places to which newly blinded persons could go to "recover confidence and competence." The first home of recovery was situated at Torquay and was named American Lodge in recognition of a munificent gift from the

British War Relief Society of the U.S.A. To this home younger people were sent because it had "all the amenities of life at a seashore resort." Because of its restful seclusion and its proximity to London, elderly people were sent to Longmeadow in Goring, the charming home of Captain Sir Beachcroft Towse, V.C., a blinded veteran of the South African War and then President of the National Institute for the Blind. The third center was Oldbury Grange, near Bridge North in the Shropshire hills. This home was where "those who love a country life find ideal conditions, with chickens and pigs, and the sounds and scents of the country-side to charm them to renewed contentment."

When it became apparent in the United States that pro-vision must be made to care for both men and women blinded in World War II, it was necessary to go before the Congress for legislation to authorize such action. The intent of the original legislation was to provide a single rehabilita-tion service which would cover all forms of disability and include all disabled in the armed services, civilian defense, and war industries. After citing the contribution that the physically handicapped could make to the war effort through rehabilitation, President Roosevelt stated in a message to the 77th Congress: "In order to secure the most effective utilization of the capabilities of the physically handicapped, it is important that a single rehabilitation service be estab-lished for both veterans and civilians."

Following that message, bills providing for a compre-hensive program for rehabilitation, including provision for the blind, both in the armed services and in civilian life, were introduced into the 77th Congress by Representative Barden of North Carolina and Senator La Follette of Wis-consin. No action was taken by the 77th Congress and similar bills were introduced at the opening of the 78th Congress. Immediate opposition to the unified program arose, and soon, under the pressure of the veterans' lobby, a bill pro-viding for service personnel alone was introduced. Promptly passed by both houses and signed by the President, it became Public Law 16 on March 24, 1943. This required a revision of the Barden-La Follette bill, deleting the armed services, and further amendment to provide for separate administration of the portions pertaining to the blind. In this revised form the legislation was passed as Public Law 113.

Public Law 16, authorizing a program of rehabilitation for those disabled while in the armed services, placed the responsibility for the establishment of this program squarely upon the Veterans Administration. This organization failed to take any action beyond the granting of pensions fixed by law to men upon severance from the services. In the meantime blinded men were being received in Army and Navy hospitals. Strange as it may seem, the best of hospitals, equal to almost any emergency, always seem to be appalled when confronted with blind patients. For example, early in the war Perkins Institution had a call from Lovell General Hospital, an Army installation at Waltham, asking if a trained attendant could be provided to care for a blinded soldier, especially one capable of feeding him. Staff members, on visiting the Hospital, with some difficulty finally persuaded the medical men that the blinded soldier could well care for himself and instead of keeping him confined with a soldier to dress and feed him that he should be sent to the Red Cross occupational therapy department and be taught to use his hands and to learn to find his way there alone.

The increasing number of blinded casualties forced the Army to provide its own program. It was early decided to concentrate all eye cases returning from the European theater at Valley Forge General Hospital, Phoenixville, Pennsylvania, and those from the Pacific area first at Letterman Hospital, San Francisco, and later at Dibble General Hospital, Palo Alto. At these centers the blinded men were placed in segregated wards and, in addition to medical care, programs of retraining were inaugurated. Workers with prior experience in work for the blind were drawn from the Army and other specialists were engaged to carry on the program of orientation, recreation, and the use of the usual tools of the sightless. Foot travel was stressed and every effort was made, as their medical and surgical care advanced, to make the men feel that they were on the road to physical adjustment and independence.

When the Army program was being planned it was expected that the Navy would coöperate. This proved not to be true, for blinded sailors were assigned to the Naval Hospital at Philadelphia, and there, in addition to medical and surgical care, a program of rehabilitation was set up for the 175 men involved, of whom 104 were marines. The program was based on two objectives, morale building and vocational orientation. To assist in attaining the latter objective, all the sailors spent two weeks at the New York Institute for the Blind, where they underwent extensive tests to determine aptitude, vocational interest, and occupational opportunities. Every effort was made to correlate the preliminary training with the possible vocational rehabilitation and other services available after discharge, through the Veterans Administration under Public Law 16. The Navy program began in January 1943 and closed in September 1946.

The training center of the Army for its blinded men was Old Farms Convalescent Hospital, opened on June 20, 1944 and continued until June 30, 1947, at Avon Old Farms, a school at Avon, Connecticut. The school plant, ruggedly built of rough stone to simulate Cotswold architecture, set in 5000 acres of land, was from the point of view of terrain, buildings, layout, and isolation, not the happiest choice but, as it was often said, "if a blind man can get about at Avon he can go anywhere." Here a program of orientation and retraining was set up under the command of Colonel Frederick Thorne, an ophthalmologist of the Army Medical Corps. In groups of 150, 850 men were processed through a course of retraining at a cost conservatively estimated at $6,000,000.

The American center might have been a St. Dunstan's, but it fell short for a number of reasons. Perhaps the results attained in England on a voluntary basis could not be expected in an Army installation, but there were few remnants of Army discipline or morale at Old Farms. A more realistic reason was that it lacked the inspiring personal leadership that prevailed at St. Dunstan's. Certainly Avon and the other centers lost an opportunity for practical help by reluctance to bring in for consultation and inspiration well-adjusted sightless men who could talk with trainees of how they had attained victory over blindness. For as a blinded veteran wrote, "An experienced blind person could have answered my questions and allayed many of my fears." And they never realized the importance of aftercare or did enough to make a good transition from the Navy or Army to the Veterans Administration.

Old Farms became too much interested in tests, not yet fully validated for the sightless, and in the psychology of a possible sixth sense or facial vision as a means of mobility. A fundamental error of the leaders was their failure to maintain continuity with the preliminary training at the Army hospitals. For example, one of the most effective developments at Valley Forge was training in the technique of foot travel by the use of a special cane. When the men reached Old Farms canes were banned and they were required to spend hours trying to avoid obstacles through facial vision. In the areas of both tests and psychology the leaders at Old Farms could have learned much from the professional teachers of the civilian blind, but they were intent on "blazing new trails."

Avon had its problems. Few of the men who came there fully realized at the time the opportunity to prepare for their new life that was available to them. Many were "fed up" with the Army and hospitals and wanted only to go home. This feeling was augmented by the fact that while in training they drew Army pay whereas upon discharge they were eligible for generous pensions. As one veteran said: "I have my $157.50 a month; what more do I need?" One parent would not allow his son to have any retraining, saying that his pension would take care of him for life and "now all that he needs is a wife." A soldier at Old Farms from the Deep South, when asked what he did before entering the Army, replied, "Nothing," and when asked what he intended to do upon discharge, replied, "The same thing."

It is easy to be critical of Old Farms, the Navy program,

and the centers at the several hospitals when viewed with "hindsight," but there is value in a realistic appraisal of what was attempted and what was accomplished. It is understood, however, that this evaluation should be of the efforts undertaken to teach young men who had suddenly been deprived of the vital gift of seeing how to face life without sight. It must also be accepted that in the area of surgical and medical care every possible effort was made to restore or conserve remaining vision. No members of the armed forces fought a more valiant battle than the ophthalmologists. A measure of their accomplishment is a report made in 1953 by Col. J. H. King, Jr., M.C., U.S.A. chief ophthalmologist, Walter Reed Hospital, that 90 percent of the soldiers blinded in World War II were rehabilitated, "one of the greatest achievements in military ophthalmology," whereas, he writes, "approximately one quarter of the blind of World War I were made self-sufficient by rehabilitation." [5]

It is true that the yardstick of this measurement was not gainful employment, the test of achievement with rehabilitation workers. It is hard to present comparable, definite statistics of accomplishment after medical care was completed because there has not been in the field of rehabilitation a study similar to that of Colonel King. In addition there are certain immeasurable factors. Generous compensation, sometimes more than the recipient might ordinarily earn, deprives many of the incentive to go out to seek a job, human nature being what it is. On the other hand, the intellectual caliber of the veterans of World War II, whose average age was twenty-two, might well make it hard for many to remain idle. In World War II 41 percent of the men in the services were high-school graduates, whereas in World War I only 4 percent had graduated from high school and 50 percent were illiterate, had little education, or were mentally retarded. If an economic survey revealed that 50 percent of the blinded servicemen of World War II are gainfully employed, that might well be considered an achievement.

Perhaps one of the most significant differences between the two wars lies in the causes of loss of sight. In World

War I nearly two-thirds were blinded by enemy action, largely through eye wounds caused by fragments of high-explosive shells and hand grenades. The other third became blind from accidents, illness, or prior ocular defects aggravated while in service. Owing to the practice in World War II of enclosing explosives, including aerial bombs, in containers of non-ferrous material, there was a decrease in eye penetration. But modern weapons have higher explosive power, so most eye damage was through concussion, causing changes in the eye, collapse, or irreparable damage from hemorrhage. Many wounds were incurred through the close-up explosion of land mines. And they brought with them added casualties through the shattering of both arms and legs. Much damage to the face called for plastic surgery. A large percentage of the 1400 blinded casualties of World War II had additional disabilities, amputations, deafness, brain damage, or debilitative disease.

The Korean conflict added its toll of over 500 blinded men, at a ratio higher than any other war; 7 percent of all casualties lost their sight. This was due to the close hand-to-hand fighting that was characteristic of that conflict. Fifty percent of the men with head wounds had eye damage. A factor not found to the same degree in earlier wars was loss of sight through malnutrition, especially among prisoners of war. It was feared that among returning prisoners there might be a resurgence of that old military ophthalmia, trachoma. But strangely there were but a few cases, most of them among the prisoners of the Communists on the Island of Koje. Among earlier prisoners of the Japanese there were practically no cases. There was no trachoma among the United States soldiers in Korea, but some appeared among other United Nations troops, especially the Ethiopians.

Upon the closing of Old Farms and the facilities at the Philadelphia Naval Hospital, care for the blinded was transferred by presidential order, May 27, 1947, to the Veterans Administration. During the last days of Avon a representative of the Veterans Administration was in residence to outline the services available under the G.I. bills. This made the transition easier. At first the Veterans Administration officers were reluctant to look with much optimism on the blinded as feasible candidates for rehabilitation. There was a definite tendency to believe that generous pensions would suffice. With further understanding of the problem, however, a better attitude was developed and soon a workable program was established.

One of the first constructive steps was to provide special training in the area of blindness for the men who were to direct rehabilitation and placement in seventy field stations. This was conducted in 1946 in coöperation with the American Foundation for the Blind. A second step was the opening on February 20, 1948 of a small center, especially for blind casualties, at Hines Veterans Hospital, near Chicago. Thus, for the first time this country had a continuing program for blinded veterans and its worth was proved when blinded personnel began to come back from the Korean conflict. Two hundred forty-nine had completed training up to December 1954. Finally a section for the blind was set up in the Department of Medicine and Surgery, whose head has authority to cut across the vertical walls of VA organization and to correlate all efforts for those without sight. This section has been able to make some revealing surveys and to lay ground work indicative of a long-time follow-up program.

The major responsibility of the Veterans Administration is the distribution of compensation as authorized by Acts of Congress. The basic law covering the present pension system was enacted July 1, 1933. Public Law 182, dated October 1, 1945, rated payments for blinded service men on the basis of the degree of their disablement. This legislation has been amended several times to increase the grants. Disability compensation for blinded veterans, according to current law (Public Law 695, dated October 1, 1954), amounts to $371 a month for anatomical loss of both eyes; $279 a month for blindness of both eyes with 5/200 central visual acuity or less (concentric contraction of the visual fields to 50 is considered no better than 5/200 central vision

for purposes of entitlement to the special monthly rate);
$329 a month for blindness in both eyes rendering the vet-
eran so helpless as to be in need of regular aid and attendance. A blinded veteran may receive an additional $47 a
month if he has suffered the loss of hearing, an arm, or a
foot, provided the total does not exceed $400 a month. Some
are confused by the distinction between the anatomical loss
of both eyes and blindness of both eyes. This phraseology was
copied from the law regarding amputees, where a distinction is readily seen. As a matter of fact, the blinded man
might well be better off, not only financially but esthetically,
with his sightless orbs replaced by the modern plastic eyes
developed during the war.

While this schedule varies according to the degree of injury, no account is taken of rank, the basis in most countries
and in the United States prior to World War I. Privates and
generals receive the same compensation for equal disability,
but officers often elect to retire on three-quarter pay. This is
deemed by many to be more democratic but it is also mani-
festly unfair if one considers cost of living in different parts
of the country and the variation of expenses involved in enabling blinded men to return to the type of life that they normally would have followed if sight had not been taken. The
young man from the South who had done nothing before
entering the Army can now continue to do the same with the
comfort of an assured check for at least $300 a month as long
as he lives. But the young man in the same group, a professional worker in the North with a wife and two children, will
have to find other means to supplement the monthly check
of the same size to attain equivalent security. Current consideration is being given to these social facts of life so that
in future legislation there may be provision for variation not
according to rank but according to the costs of restoring a
man to the standards by which he would have lived if his sight
had not been taken while he was in the service of his country.

In any consideration of financial aid for the blind there are
certain aspects that must be stated. In the first place there is
considered to be a difference between payments to civilians

and to the war blinded. In practically all countries payment to civilians is designed to offset the recognized additional costs imposed by loss of sight. It is usually revocable, generally based on the factor of need, and may be reduced as the blind person's income increases. The money paid to a man blinded in the service of his country is considered compensation for that loss, whereas the term pension is used to designate the benefit for disability not due to service. In European countries financial aid is referred to as reparation or indemnity. The monetary compensation is for life and is not reduced when a veteran is gainfully employed. General Omar N. Bradley, when Administrator of Veteran's Affairs, pointed out that compensation had no relation to things past but, rather, had been created to assist the disabled veteran in the future. It is society's way of paying for sight lost in war.

In 1955 the United States through the Veterans Administration was making payments to slightly more than 5000 persons with severe eye disabilities, as follows:

	Percentage of disability				
	100	90	80	70	Total
Korea	270	37	78	141	526
World War II	1,724	216	471	946	3357
World War I	773	55	65	238	1131
Spanish-American War	8	0	1	1	10
					5024

Assuming an average payment of $300 a month, the total cost of war-incurred blindness in this country amounts to over $1,500,000 a month or an annual toll approaching $20,000,000. Beyond that figure, however, is a sizable amount paid for eye disablement not within the definition of blindness, which for compensation is 5/200 and for rehabilitation benefits 20/200.

A significant factor revealed in these figures is the advance in the number of those who are now receiving compensation over those blinded in active service. In World War I the number who lost their sight in conflict was approximately 300. Now there are over 1000 veterans of that war receiving compensation for blindness. The sharp ascent following war is shown in the total of 3357 veterans of World War II now receiving aid, whereas at the time of the armistice the number of blinded casualties was listed as 1400. And the slow decline of pensioners is indicated by the fact that the Veterans Administration is still carrying on its rolls ten men blinded as a consequence of service in the Spanish-American War. It is possible that the peak of blind casualties of the two world wars may reach 10,000, especially if the Veterans Administration continues to accept responsibility for nonservice-incurred loss of sight, and society will be making payments for the toll of war for fifty years more.

One of the aftermaths of war that often has social consequences is the formation of veterans groups. In this generation they have become potent social forces in practically all countries. Most of these organizations were intended originally to continue fellowships closely woven in war, but many have become motivated by a desire to seek compensation for the sacrifices made by their members through war service. As eye casualties generally involve lifetime disablement, the war blinded in nearly all countries have developed their own organizations and in varying degrees they have become pressure groups. In England and the British Commonwealth there is not the same need for an independent group because of the comprehensive program of St. Dunstan's and that organization's active concern for the aftercare of its members following both wars.

After World War I an attempt was made to found a society of blinded veterans in the United States, but it soon folded, partly because of poor organization, partly because of the small number involved, but perhaps chiefly because this country made good provision for its blind casualties through compensation and opportunity for rehabilitation. In addition the blind shared in the benefits secured by the larger and all-inclusive associations of veterans. The need for organization of the blinded veterans at the close of World War II was made apparent by the confusion as to how a program of rehabilitation was to be promoted. To obtain the services to which they felt entitled, those who had given their sight in war soon determined that through association they could best help themselves.

This feeling led to the formation of the Blinded Veterans Association in March 1945. Its motivating force was self-help and that form of support which comes through sharing mutual experiences. Membership in the Association indicates not only a desire to live up to its standards but also to help others do so. The "playing up" of men who have achieved success is a positive approach new in veteran propaganda. B.V.A. has never become a pressure group, although it has not hesitated to set forth the claims of the blinded for rehabilitation and other forms of self-help. For if, wrote Lloyd Greenwood, "it can be established that the benefits provided for the veteran have eased and expedited his adjustment to the conditions of blindness, perhaps all of America's blind may profit in the future." [6] The Association maintains an office for its elected secretary, holds annual conventions, and publishes a very readable monthly magazine.

It is necessary to turn to Europe to find highly organized, aggressive associations of the war blinded that have lifted their benefits far above those provided for the civilian sightless. Nearly all have affiliation with the powerful World Veterans Federation, which has 28,000,000 members. Perhaps one of the strongest groups is the Italian Union of the War Blind, which has a magnificent center in Rome and large workshops in both Rome and Florence. Full employment is assured through work provided by the Army and other government agencies. The Italian Union is now using its strong influence to have a part in organizations for the civilian blind. Legislation is being pressed to require all agencies for the blind to have on their boards of directors at least one blind member chosen by the Union. Blinded veterans in Germany organized in 1916, and in 1932 had more than 3000 members. In 1934 Hitler provided a building in Berlin for their use, with a museum, a braille library, and living quarters for visiting blind veterans.

The Union of the French War Blind, founded in 1918,

while stressing the development of social life among its members, never loses sight of financial compensation. It maintains three homes which can be used by members for "health or holiday" and provides scholarships for the children of its members. In the area of financial aid the French Union has finally attained a security unequaled by the civilian blind in any country and indicative of why leaders of the civilian blind are seeking to bring their benefits up to the level attained by the war blinded. Henri Amblard, at the Assembly of the World Council for the Welfare of the Blind held in Paris in August 1954, stated it clearly: "Men from the two World Wars have joined forces at the head of the Association and recently we obtained a guarantee which may interest any among the blind that are in need of pensions or allowances. It has been agreed that there shall be a constant ratio between a civil servant's salary and our pensions. This law has come into force, so we need no longer make repeated demands in order that our pensions may maintain relative value."

15 WHO ARE THE BLIND?

INCREASING provision of economic compensation for the visually handicapped and the growing plans for the conquest of blindness make it imperative to know who are entitled to the modern programs of help and how large the field of need is. Fundamental questions today are: Who are the blind, and what ratio of the world's population do they represent? Securing answers to these questions would seem to be a relatively simple matter. As a matter of fact it is very complex. This is because there is no common agreement as to who is to be considered blind and who is not. And until that is determined the extent of blindness in the community or in the world cannot be ascertained. Many existing statistics in this field have no validity because of differing definitions as they are applied today to that segment of society which labors under visual disability.

Turning to the dictionary, one learns that the adjective "blind" means "sightless"; that is, without sight. On the basis of that, it is assumed that a blind person is one who cannot see. So it was in the ancient world. But that is not so in modern society. Today there are included among the blind not only those within the dictionary definition, but also a very large number of persons whose sight is so restricted that it constitutes not only a visual disability but also an economic liability. This places within the modern category of the blind a seemingly increasing number of persons, and establishes blindness as a major social problem which even in this day is not intelligently understood or efficiently handled.

Before proceeding to the consideration of a definition of

blindness under modern conditions, it may be desirable to give some thought to the sense of sight, the lack of which, and, in these days, certain limitations of which, constitute legal blindness. In its simplest terms, sight is created by the admission of rays of light to the organ of sight, the eye. Light travels in a straight line until deflected by an object. In the eye, the lens deflects the divergent rays of light so that they may come to a focus on the retina, the rear inner wall of the eye.

While the eye is a marvelous organ, in modern man it is revealed as far from perfect. Only one or two in a hundred people have theoretically ideal eyes and in practically every other eye the distance between the lens and the retina varies from the ideal. This affects vision. If the distance is shorter than normal, the projected rays come to a focus beyond the retina, and if the condition is severe it must be corrected by a convex lens. If the distance is longer than normal, the point of focus falls short of the retina and a concave lens must be employed for correction.

The eye, however, has a marvelous power of accommodation whereby it is able to overcome all but severe deviations from the norm; therefore not all persons have to wear glasses, the modern medium for correction. Those whose eyes focus beyond the retina—and they represent more than two-thirds of the inhabitants of America and Britain—are considered "far sighted," that is, they can see distant objects more clearly than objects close at hand. Technically, their condition is described as hyperopia. Those whose eyes focus short of the retina are better equipped for close work than for distant vision and their condition is known as myopia.

There is another error of refraction found in many eyes called "astigmatism" which is the failure of the eye structure to focus all of the rays of light at the same point owing to an irregularity in the curved surface of the cornea, the front covering of the eyeball. This condition may occur with either far or near sight. Because of these and many other errors and imperfections, John Milton out of his blindness might well ask:

Why was the sight
To such a tender ball as th' eye confin'd?
So obvious and so easie to be quench't,
And not as feeling through all parts diffus'd,
That she might look at will through every pore? [1]

Confining sight to "such a tender ball" as the eye, however, has advantages. It is compact, its mechanics are easily understood, and its efficiency can be measured. In the effort to define blindness the possibility of measurement is of prime importance, especially when it transcends the definition of the dictionary and involves physical defects and refractive errors as well as the degree of intelligent interpretation of the images cast upon the retina.

The fact must not be overlooked that two other organs function in making sight meaningful: the optic nerve and the brain. The eye may be perfect and ready to perform with full efficiency but yet give no visual experience. This is because the optic nerve is not functioning and therefore the visual image never reaches the centers of the brain which interpret and make it meaningful. High in any list of causes of blindness is "atrophy of the optic nerve," a blanket term covering a multitude of possible defects in the nervous system between the eye and the brain center. Regardless of the specific cause, if the optic nerve is atrophied, the person cannot see, even with a perfect eye, and therefore is blind.

The third organ in the science of sight and often the most important one is the brain, the interpreter of the light rays that focus on the retina and there give rise to the nerve impulses that are transmitted through the optic nerve. In studies of blindness, not enough attention has been paid to this center of interpretation. In these days when those with some useful vision are included within the category of the blind, their ability to interpret what they see may well be the determining factor in their classification as blind or sighted. For as someone has said: "A first-class brain can make good use of an imperfect eye." [2]

The mental capacity to use effectively the remaining vision is quite as important in determining blindness from the social point of view as is the physical measurement of visual acuity. Is society today including within the modern category of blindness many persons who through their own intellectual ability or through reëducation could be lifted above the necessity of blind relief? Is the seemingly increasing number of blind persons due to the present tendency to define blindness in too generous terms?

Of course, these questions apply only to those with some usable vision. In the days when blind persons were considered to be the completely sightless, there were not as many forms of occupation that required perfect vision. The ancient world called for little close work such as the modern world requires of its office and machine workers. And there were no automobiles to make the roads hazardous to those with restricted vision. Only those who could not see at all were made a class apart and to the old world they were, as Europeans still say, "the blind." Society recognized them as such and pictured them as beggars sitting at the gates of the temples or as blind bards making their way from town to town.

The present social practice of considering limited vision an economic handicap and an intellectual barrier is a relatively recent phenomenon. While many factors conspired to focus attention on the restrictions of partial sight, the invention of printing and the production of books precipitated the whole matter. People wanted to read the new books and many found out that they could not. Dr. Arnold Sorsby in his *History of Ophthalmology* indicates that the desire to read was a potent factor in making persons with impaired vision conscious of their loss. He states that a social urge caused by the spread of literacy and the development of newspapers and literature motivated people to seek ways of improving sight so that more of them could read. The early answer to this problem was the use of spectacles whose lenses could correct the errors of shortsightedness, farsightedness, and astigmatism.

Legend claims that eyeglasses were invented by Saint Jerome (347–420), which might well be true, since he was the most notable student of Didymus (308–395), the great blind scholar of Alexandria. The claim inscribed on a tomb in a church in Florence, however, should not be overlooked: "Here lies Salvino degli Armatis, the inventor of spectacles. Died 1317. May God pardon his sins." No matter who invented them, spectacles were known in both China and Europe in the thirteenth century and by the sixteenth century were in common use.

Roger Bacon (1214–1294?) is said to have recommended the use of convex lenses to correct the failing sight of the aged (presbyopia) in 1268, and as early as the sixteenth century concave lenses were used for the correction of myopia. It was not until 1807 that Thomas Young (1773–1829), English physicist and physician, discovered that errors of refraction leading to astigmatism could be corrected by glasses, and the invention of bifocals in 1784 is attributed to Benjamin Franklin. All of these discoveries were based on the much earlier claim of the German astronomer and mathematician, Johannes Kepler (1571–1630), that "Images were painted on the retina and that the crystalline lens refracted the rays of light and brought them to a focal point." At the end of the sixteenth century, Kepler "gave an almost complete account of the way in which rays of light are bent within the eye and how this results in the formation of an image on the retina." [3]

From the earliest use of glasses, ways had to be found to determine the most helpful types of lenses, and at first the tests were very crude. In England, and probably in other countries, charlatans conducted what today would be called a racket. Going from town to town with a bagful of glasses, they tried different lenses on persons eager to read until the type in the book in hand was clearly focused, probably more by anticipation than by actual correction. In 1843, the first scientific trial case was introduced. It consisted of accurately ground lenses which were tried on the patient until the right combination was found. In the same year, Heinrich Küchler (1811–1873) developed a series of lines of letters for testing near vision. In 1851, Eduard von Jaeger (1818–1884) in Vienna produced his twenty sizes of reading type which are still used for testing vision at short distances, although there are modern adaptations whose ratings correlate with those of Snellen for long distances.

In 1851, Hermann L. F. von Helmholtz (1821–1894), a German pioneer in physiological optics, invented an ophthalmoscope, and six years later, Dr. Albrecht von Graefe (1828–1870), a German ophthalmologist whose father was a pioneer in plastic surgery, began to put it to practical use. Wherever these instruments were used, different tests were developed. "Just as formerly," wrote Herman Snellen, "every town and province desired a different coinage and standard of measurement, so it appears that every school of ophthalmology must boast of its own ophthalmoscopes and its own visual tests." [4] To avoid this confusion, Dr. von Graefe asked a Dutch ophthalmologist to put eye testing on a scientific basis.

The Dutch ophthalmologist selected to establish a scientific measurement of vision was Herman Snellen. Born in Zeist, Holland, in 1834, the son of a physician, he received his medical degree in 1857 at the University of Utrecht. Remaining in that community until his death in 1908, he became in 1858 attached to the Netherlands Hospital for Eye Patients and devoted himself to the field of ophthalmology, where he attained great distinction, especially for operations on the eye. In 1877, he became Professor of Ophthalmology at the University of Utrecht, serving in that capacity until 1899. In 1884, Dr. Snellen became director of the Netherlands Hospital, continuing until 1903. He succeeded the famous Dr. Franz Cornelius Donders (1818–1889), who introduced the present type of ophthalmoscope.

In undertaking his task, Snellen drew heavily on the achievements of his predecessor Dr. Donders, undoubtedly the greatest authority on geometric optics at that time and the first to separate clearly the errors of refraction from those of accommodation. Donders also proved that the antithesis of myopia (nearsightedness) was hyperopia (farsightedness) and not presbyopia; up to that time it had been associated with the loss of vision in old age, thereby accounting for the anomaly known as the "old sight of young people." According to Dr. Sorsby, "It was largely the work of Donders that made the problems of refraction and the rational use of glasses part of the ophthalmic creed." [5]

Snellen's competence in ophthalmology and his sound training in optics under Donders made him the ideal person to develop from Donders' complicated scientific formulas (in which it is said every symbol of the Greek alphabet was used) a practical way not only to determine a patient's visual acuity but also to find the correct lenses needed to compensate for refractive errors. In simple terms, Snellen's problem was to find the correction needed to make abnormal eyes see clearly and, with those of limited vision, to ascertain how much they are able to see with maximum correction.

"Visual acuity," Snellen wrote, "is measured in the same way as the tactile sensitivity is determined, that is, by the minimum distance at which two simultaneous impressions give rise to two independent sensations." [6] His immediate task was to determine the minimum distance at which symbols could be seen clearly. To make this measurement, Snellen changed from the usual charts of readable text to the use of single letters. For the major symbol, he selected *E* because it most closely simulated the three parallel lines used by Donders in his studies of optics.

To determine the size of the letter, a visual angle of five minutes was chosen. For the normal eye to see the *E* clearly within that arc at 200 feet, the letter had to be 3.48 inches square. When its three arms with the two interspaces were divided equally, each printed line subtended an angle of one minute. From that start and on the same principle, Snellen added ten rows of the more readily distinguishable letters, with those of the last row 0.18 inches square. The letters of each row were of a size that, subtending the visual angle of five minutes, they could be read clearly at these distances: 100, 70, 60, 40, 30, 20, 15, and 10 feet.

Today the chart devised by Dr. Snellen for the determination of the acuteness of vision is to be found in eye hospitals in all parts of the world. For modern testing in the ophthalmologist's office, it is placed, well illuminated, at a distance of 20 feet, with the 20-foot line of letters at eye level, since normal eyes are practically at rest when viewing objects at that distance. Usually the tester will begin with the largest letter and work downward until the testee reaches the line of letters that are beyond his ability to read readily. A person with normal vision should be able to distinguish clearly the 20-foot line at a distance of 20 feet, and if so, his visual acuity is rated as 20/20. If he cannot read clearly the letters of the 70-foot line, he is rated 20/70 and comes within the category called the partially seeing. If he can see only the large letter *E*, his visual acuity is 20/200, and he is on the threshold of being considered blind according to the present American definition.

It must be understood that these ratings are not to be interpreted as fractions but as scientific measurements of acuteness of vision, nor should they be confused with measurements of the efficient use of whole or partial sight. They conform to Snellen's formula: $V = d/D$, in which V means visual acuity, d is the distance of the person from the chart, and D is the distance at which the letters are clearly read by persons with normal vision. For example, 20/200 does not mean, as many think, that a person with that acuity is visually restricted to 10 percent of the effective use of normal sight. As a matter of fact he has a visual efficiency of 20 percent.

Since Snellen's time, ophthalmologists have become increasingly concerned over the ability of people with impaired vision to use efficiently their remaining sight. Whereas visual acuity is the exact measurement of remaining sight, visual efficiency is defined as the competence of the eyes to accomplish their physiological purposes. That competence, as a percentage, has been related to the Snellen ratings by the Section on Ophthalmology of the American Medical Association and revised in 1955 as follows: [7]

Snellen Rating of Visual Acuity	Percent Central Visual Efficiency	Percent Loss of Visual Efficiency
20/20	100	0
20/40	85	15
20/50	75	25
20/80	60	40
20/100	50	50
20/200	20	80

This table and much of what has been written in this chapter so far may seem to concern, not blind people, but rather those of limited vision. In a way this is true. But in the effort to determine who is to be considered blind, there is no argument about those who meet the dictionary definition of "sightless." There is, however, considerable room for argument as to where the line is to be drawn in the field of limited vision. How much loss of sight makes people physical, educational, economic, and social problems? What other factors should be included in a definition that will be fair both to the persons physically involved and to those who assume social responsibility for them? Certainly, as has been pointed out, the mental ability to use limited vision is a factor as important as the most scientific measurement of visual acuity.

In determining visual acuity, Dr. Snellen was the first to acknowledge the limitations of his tests in the lower range of useful sight. "When visual acuity is greatly reduced," he wrote, "it is not possible to measure with the same precision," [8] and he suggested testing with fingers held apart against a dark background, which a person with normal vision should be able to count at 1 meter. This is the method devised by the French physician, Armand Trousseau (1801–1867), and the one still largely used in Europe for the determination of blindness and frequently in this country for quick screening.

With this method, a person is considered blind who cannot count fingers at 1 meter or who, as it is rated, has a visual acuity of 1/60. For the record, it should be stated that the Snellen computations were originally in meters but have been cited here in feet because Americans are more accustomed to expressing the measurements in that way. For comparison, 60 meters is approximately 200 feet and 20 feet nearly equals 6 meters, so that perfect vision in meters would be 6/6 and in feet 20/20. The American definition of blindness, 20/200, expressed in meters would be 6/60. Comparing that with the English rating of 3/60 and the European standard of 1/60, one sees the wide variation in definitions of blindness, which cause unfairness in assigning benefits and confusion in evaluating statistics.

Although the mechanics of testing visual acuity are now well established, there is still no common agreement as to who is blind and who is not. The problem has been referred to the World Health Organization and thought given to the matter has reached a point where

It was agreed that a definition which would be internationally accepted should:
(a) Assure that all persons whose visual handicap is such that they are in need of special services have an equal right and access to such services;
(b) Insure that persons not entitled to such services do not benefit from them and are not considered as being blind; and,
(c) Make it possible, when programs for the blind are being developed, to assess the extent of the problem.[9]

Until this referral to the WHO, practically all definitions have been based on national needs and methods. In the United States, each state had its own definition until 1935, when the adoption of the Social Security Act with provision for aid to the blind required some national standard for its administration. Two years prior to that, the American Medical Association's section on ophthalmology had recommended, not a uniform definition, but definitions of several grades of blindness. Economic blindness was described as "the inability to do any kind of work for which sight is essential." This was explained as meaning that "objects can be recognized only when brought within one-tenth of the distance at which they can be recognized with standard vision. Such vision in the better eye when corrected with the best possible glass would be recorded as less than 0.1 or 6/60 or 20/200 or an equally disabling loss of the visual field."

When states set up their plans to implement the benefits of the new Social Security legislation, the Bureau of Public Assistance recommended the definition of economic blindness proposed by the American Medical Association, with stress placed on ophthalmic measurements. This led to the

adoption by most states of the now generally prevailing definition fixing the line determining blindness arbitrarily at
20/200 in terms of the Snellen Chart. In doing this, the flexible aspect of the original American Medical Association
definition was lost and the opportunity to exercise judgment
as to the person's ability to use residual sight was ignored.

It is now being recognized that defining blindness in terms
of ophthalmic measurements, even when most scientifically
determined, is not always accurate or fair. In the first place,
a measurement of visual acuity attained on the basis of the
Snellen Chart is not adequate, a fact which Dr. Snellen
pointed out, for that formula applies chiefly to distant vision
and is more accurate in the upper range of sight. In many
cases, near vision is the critical factor, certainly for admission
to schools for the blind. In arriving at an acceptable definition, near vision must be given the same scientific consideration that is now given to distant vision.

A second factor that must not be overlooked is the ability
of a person to use his residual sight, or visual efficiency. Too
many visually handicapped persons are classified as blind on
the basis of the Snellen tests who by "using their brains" need
not be considered blind. As previously quoted, "a first-class
brain can make very good use of an imperfect eye." A third
factor that is fundamentally related is the need of more consideration of the kind of work that can be successfully performed with limited vision. More effort to find such fields of
occupation might considerably reduce the number now considered economically blind. The wide variance to be found
in these human factors militates against the effectiveness of
determining blindness by ophthalmic measurements and calls
for a more flexible type of definition.

England recognized the importance of a flexible definition
when in 1920 it defined as blind a person "unable to perform
any work for which eyesight is essential." Later, when opthal-
mic measurements were set up, provision was made to weigh
the person's ability to use his residual sight and to consider
how much vision his work required. In ophthalmic terms,
England now considers as blind a person whose visual acuity

on the Snellen Chart does not exceed 3/60, which is one-half the maximum prescribed in the United States. But in the area between 3/60 and 6/60, the benefits available to blind persons may be granted if personal factors make it seem desirable. It is interesting to note that the British are becoming more generous in their consideration of the intervening group, for the proportion receiving benefits has advanced from 4.1 percent in 1934 to 22.6 in 1950.

In working toward an adequate definition of blindness, consideration must be given to (1) the actual amount of residual sight in terms of both distant and near vision, (2) the extent to which it can be used without detrimental effects, (3) the ability of the person to use efficiently his remaining vision, and (4) the amount of sight that is essential for the person involved to earn his livelihood or to acquire an education. These requirements presume that every provision for sight restoration or correction have been explored and exercised. Perhaps no one definition of blindness can ever be adequate and the recommendation of the American Medical Society in 1933 that there be several definitions may have to be accepted.

The World Council for the Welfare of the Blind at its assembly in Paris in August 1954, after careful consideration of the need for uniformity, proposed three criteria for defining blindness: (1) total absense of sight; (2) visual acuity not exceeding 3/60 or 10/200 in the better eye with correction; and (3) serious visual limitation up to an arc subtending 20°. The Council stressed the 3/60 requirement as basic and members were instructed to urge their governments and agencies to adopt that as an important first step. It was the opinion of this group representing over thirty nations that agreement on such a definition would help open the way toward compilation of accurate statistical knowledge on which relief and rehabilitation programs must be based.

16 THE EXTENT OF
BLINDNESS

IN setting sights for the conquest of blindness, it is necessary to know its extent as well as the range of the disability. It has been pointed out that the term "blind" has many meanings and that there is still confusion as to who is blind and who is not. Great progress has been made in understanding the science of sight and in determining visual acuity. Knowledge of the causes of loss of sight is constantly widening and new cures and preventive measures are being developed. The immediate and most pressing need is to arrive at a definition of blindness universally acceptable and, by applying it, to find out the extent of the problem in terms of both disability and the number of persons involved.

In the previous chapter, it was indicated that perhaps the earliest attempt at a practical way of determining who is blind was made by the French ophthalmologist, Armand Trousseau. About 1850, he defined blindness as "the inability to count fingers at a distance of 1 meter in any circumstances." While many countries still adhere to the distance aspect of Trousseau's definition, other countries have undertaken to control the "circumstances" under which the measurement is made.

Norway, for example, states that a blind person is one who "cannot count fingers in a good light against a dark background." Italy, however, is less explicit, defining the near-blind as those "unable to count fingers at a reasonable distance." India recommended that "A person unable to count the fingers of a hand held up at a yard's distance should be considered blind." Trousseau's definition was accepted at the Australia Medical Congress in 1934 and is still in use in many other countries, including China, Germany, Hungary, Poland, and Sweden. While lacking scientific accuracy, this test is easy and practical in application and serves effectively for screening and preliminary testing.

One of the earliest reasons for a more accurate definition of blindness was to determine the necessity for financial aid to those unable to work. Many definitions have that purpose primarily in mind, even though the methods of measuring the loss of sight may differ. For example, a definition early incorporated in The Workman's Compensation Act in Pennsylvania stated that "a person incapable of reading the 200-foot line at 20 feet was considered blind in the sense that he was not fit to do any kind of work requiring vision." In Greece, "A person is considered blind who has 1/25 visual acuity, or impairment of vision great enough to prevent the handicapped from pursuing the type of work which he would have done under normal conditions." Austria reports 1/25 normal vision as economically worthless, and Denmark states that "adults with visual power not more than 4/60 or having vision of no practical value are blind."

Other countries base their definitions on the ability or lack of ability of a blind person to get about. France defines as blind "a person with 1/20 vision, or with weakening of the vision carried to such a point that those affected cannot get about alone," while in the Netherlands, a blind person is one "not in a position to go out into the street without a guide." Finland and Switzerland consider as blind those "who cannot find their way in unfamiliar surroundings." The little colony of Nigeria throws the burden of determining a person's blindness upon his associates with this definition: "So blind as to be recognized as blind by one's fellows."

Germany in the 1925 census makes the same point with considerable amplification: "In addition to the totally blind, all persons whose sight is so bad that even equipped with spectacles they cannot find their way about in places unfamiliar to them, or count at a distance of 1 meter the outstretched fingers of a hand against a dark background, shall be considered blind. Persons who are blind in one eye only are not regarded as blind." The United States' definition for the census of 1920—"cannot see well enough to read even with the aid of glasses"—also needed amplification. The instructions, therefore, told enumerators to make some allowance for infants who had not yet learned to read, and for illiterates to be included if they could not "see enough to read if they knew how to read."

The United States is said to have the only definition of blindness expressed in ophthalmic terms: "A person shall be considered blind who has a visual acuity not exceeding 20/200 in the better eye with correcting lenses, or visual acuity greater than 20/200 but with a limitation in the fields of vision such that the widest diameter of the visual fields subtends an angle no greater than 20°." This definition is now generally accepted for admission to schools for the blind, for benefits under rehabilitation, and for financial aid under Social Security.

The British like to refer to the practicality of their definition: "A person who is so blind as to be unable to perform any work for which eyesight is essential." It is interesting to note, however, that the Section of Ophthalmology of the Royal Society of Medicine considered it advisable to supplement this general definition by numerical standards expressing degrees of blindness, pointing out that "experience shows that persons whose visual acuity is below 3/60 Snellen are usually unable to perform work requiring eyesight, while those with vision better than 6/60 are usually able to perform some such work. Persons with intermediate degrees may or may not be able; much depends on intelligence and bodily strength and much on the nature of the blindness."

Dr. Arnold Sorsby, the English authority on blindness and its causes, does not feel that fixing the point at 3/60 is substantiated by enough investigation in industry but admits that it is a considerable advance over the Trousseau definition of 1/60 though still a long way from the United States standard of 20/200 and the equivalent Canadian standard of 6/60. He then poses a pertinent question: "Is the American standard of 20/200 (or approximately 6/60) too high or is the British standard of 3/60 too low?" [1]

A general summary of the attempt to define blindness in ophthalmic terms of visual acuity indicates that the maximum vision for one rated as blind is 20/200 (feet) or 6/60 (meters). There are, however, several other variable factors as, for example, the present British interpretation that those with vision between "3/60 and 6/60 may be classified as blind or not blind according to fullness or restrictions of the field of vision." In defining restrictions in the field of vision, social agencies in the United States have set an arc of 20°, and Canada of 10°, in which there is no limit in acuity; that is, a person may have perfect sight within the prescribed arc, but because of the restricted field he will be rated as blind. The United States Navy, however, in its definition, restricts the arc to 15°, while the United States Army in some regulations considers blindness as 5/200 in acuity, which is less than the British acuity. These factors pose elements of flexibility that hamper a rigid definition in ophthalmic terms. The attainment of uniformity is further handicapped by the possibility of maladministration of tests or faulty response on the part of the persons being tested.

Coming to the attempt to ascertain how many blind people there are in the world, the confusing definitions and the varying standards create a problem twice confounded. For the validity of statistics regarding the extent of blindness depends on the uniformity of the definition of what constitutes blindness and the reliability of the methods of ascertainment. It has already been pointed out that there is no uniform definition of blindness. That leaves methods of ascertainment to be considered. The League of Nations' study of blindness made in 1929 reports: "Experience shows that it is very difficult, if not impossible, to secure complete statistics. There are three ways in which such statistics can be, theoretically speaking, compiled. One is by compulsory notification of blindness; two, by the census; and three, by special registration of the blind." [2]

"Compulsory notification of blindness by medical practitioners of blind persons," the League of Nations Report stated, "has not, so far as it is known, been attempted in any country." Since then, certain states within the United States, including Massachusetts, have passed legislation requiring notification, but considerable doubt exists as to full compliance with the law. It is a method, however, that should be promoted, for beyond its statistical value it does bring to the attention of the proper authorities blind children or blinded persons for whom some medical care, rehabilitation, or assistance may be provided in the early stages when most needed. It will also make the medical practitioners more conscious of the social importance of blindness. While this method would give reliable information as far as it goes, it is doubtful whether it will ever go far enough to be the sole method of ascertainment.

The United States was the first country to try to enumerate the blind through the census, beginning in 1830. One hundred years later, this method was given up as unreliable. Other countries have had the same experience owing to the inability of the enumerators to determine who should be listed as blind and the reluctance of many families to reveal blind members. Generally, census figures have been considered so far below the estimated number of blind persons as to have little or no value. More recent analysis, however, seems to indicate that the census enumerators were the innocent victims of the confusion caused by the varying definitions of blindness.

The United States Census of 1930, the last to include the blind, listed 63,489 blind persons. It was generally felt by workers in this field that there were many more blind people than that. The census of 1920 had reported 57,444 as blind, but the special report entitled *The Blind in the United States; 1920,* arrived at the conclusion that an "estimate of between 74,500 and 76,600 as the totally blind population of 1920 is a reasonably close approximation to the truth." [3] Careful statistics gathered a few years later by several states sustained the incompleteness of the census figure.

The New York State Commission for the Blind claimed that the correct number of blind persons in that state was 90 percent greater than the number returned in the census. In Colorado in 1922, pensions were being given to 44 percent more blind persons than the census enumerators reported. Another interesting illustration of the difficulty in securing an accurate count is found in the United States Census of 1880, which reported 48,929 blind persons. This was double the number enrolled in the report of ten years previous, which was 20,220. Workers for the blind were concerned that blindness might have doubled in a decade. A possible explanation for the doubling, however, was the fact that enumerators received a bonus of five cents for each case of blindness reported!

In Germany, the last census of the blind was taken in 1925. This indicated a total of 36,769 people, or 59 per 100,000 population, on the basis of counting fingers at 1 meter. The returns, however, were considered so inadequate that census enumeration was discontinued. At the Oxford Conference in 1949, France offered "no figures on the ground that census returns are unreliable," but indicated that there were approximately 42,000 blind persons of whom only 22,000 were within the definition of the law of 1945, that is, 1/20.

The Union of South Africa gave up the enumeration of persons with deformities because "the information obtained in this report is so incomplete as to be entirely misleading . . . less blind children of school-going age were registered in the whole Union than the number of children actually attending a school at one center." In Great Britain, when 26,-336 were reported in 1911, "it was decided (1921) to omit the inquiry as to 'infirmities,' included in previous censuses, in view of the generally recognized fact that reliable information upon these subjects cannot be expected in returns made by or on behalf of the individuals afflicted."

Since 1921, the census enumerators, at least in England, have found a champion. Dr. Sorsby in his *Causes of Blindness in England and Wales* points out that "the definition of blindness has become less rigid than in days gone by," that

"earlier there was a general acceptance of Trousseau's definition, which implied vision of 1/60 (Snellen) or less," and
that "the census figures were based on an even more stringent
definition." Using a more liberal definition suggested by the
Royal Society of Medicine in 1915, a register of the blind was
taken in 1919, which totaled 77,390 persons. But only 25,840,
or 30 percent, conform to the definition used in enumerating
the 26,336 reported in the 1911 census. "Contrary to the general belief," states Dr. Sorsby, "the census figures are, therefore, not grossly inaccurate for the degree of blindness ('total
blindness') they sought to establish. In any case, it is clear
that the increase in the numbers of the registered blind is
largely consequent on a change in definition." [4] This is undoubtedly true in the United States and in other countries.

The most reliable and accurate method of ascertaining the
number of blind persons is through registration, provided
there is a commonly accepted definition. Dr. Sorsby points
out the difference a definition can make. The register in
England in 1948 of 76,009 is based on a definition of 3/60
or less, plus a limited number up to 6/60, making a ratio of
175 per 100,000. If the definition were more stringent, covering total blindness and only light perception, or 1/50, the
ratio would be 60 per 100,000, conforming to the reports to
the Oxford Conference of several European countries. If the
limit of vision were increased to 6/60, "the rate of blindness
would rise to about 250, a figure in line with experience in
Canada and the United States." [5]

Neither Canada nor the United States reported at Oxford
a ratio as high as that quoted by Dr. Sorsby. Canada indicated
an incidence of 150 based on its 18,200 persons registered as
having visual acuity of 6/60 or under. The United States reported 230,354 with 6/60 or 20/200, making a ratio of 175.
While the ratio in the United States is the same as that in
England, the definition on which the estimate is made is
much more generous. If the English definition of 3/60 were
used in the United States, the total number and the incidence
would both be considerably less, perhaps as much as 25 percent, whereas if the rigid European definition, that is 1/60,

were applied in this country, the story here would be quite different and the number classified as blind would be reduced perhaps by another 25 percent—another illustration of how meaningless statistics of blindness are because of the difference of definitions.

In addition to the three ways of ascertaining the extent of blindness suggested in the League of Nations Report, and perhaps because of their inadequacy, another method is now being widely accepted. This is to estimate according to an accepted definition the number of blind persons in any area. In many countries there is no other way, and in some, guessing is perhaps a more accurate term than estimating. For to have any validity, an estimate must be based on a core of basic facts and there must be able competence in applying them. Without doubt, this method of determining the number of blind persons has reached a high degree of validity in the United States, where it has produced statistics regarding blindness that are far more reliable than those obtained through the census and more comprehensive than any available through state registers.

In 1929, a Committee on the Statistics of the Blind was sponsored by the American Foundation for the Blind and the National Society for the Prevention of Blindness. After determining and recommending the definition now generally accepted in this country, the Committee turned its attention to finding out how many persons fell within it. Dr. Ralph G. Hurlin, a social statistician and now vice-president of the Russell Sage Foundation, served as chairman of the Committee from 1930 until 1955. Much of the reliability of the estimates made has been due to his competency in this area of statistics and his careful studies in the field of blindness.

After a number of surveys and studies, the Committee arrived at a formula that, when applied to the population of a state, indicated the number of blind persons resident therein. "Two basic assumptions were made in arriving at the estimated rates of prevalence of blindness," Dr. Hurlin wrote, "A. That the rates will vary from state to state, and B. that the rate for each state will be determined chiefly by the composition of its population with respect to age, race, and state public health standards." [6] The varying state rates were predicated on an analysis of the three factors listed in the second assumption.

Of these three· factors, age and race were readily determined statistically, but the third, public health standards, was not as easy to evaluate and rate. In his latest study, Dr. Hurlin felt that the infant death rate of a state represented the best gauge of its public health standards, for when the infant death rate is low, he claims, good health services are indicated. This principle applies generally in all states. Therefore the infant death rate was adopted as the best index of the state's public health standards.

Old age was considered critical because it is well established that a high prevalence of loss of sight is now found among aged people. The importance of the racial factor is based on the knowledge, gained from earlier studies, that among nonwhites blindness is from two to three times as frequent as among white persons. This is not due to any racial characteristics but reflects the lower economic and health standards, especially among Negroes in the South and Indians in the West.

These three factors were further balanced through a system of weights designed to cover known variations in the different states. When the data for each state were gathered, carefully weighed, and reduced to a percentage, this was applied to the actual statistics of one state. For the most recent study, North Carolina was selected because it has a competent State Commission for the Blind with a large staff, which had computed by actual count the number of blind persons as of June 30, 1952. The application of this formula to the population figures of all states as of July 1, 1952 led the Committee on the Statistics of the Blind to announce in March 1953 that its estimate of the number of blind persons in this country was 308,419, making a ratio of 198 per 100,000 population.

This estimate is larger than those previously reported by the Committee. In 1940, the estimated total was 230,354 blind persons, or a prevalence rate of 175 per 100,000 population. These were the figures reported at the Oxford Conference and previously quoted herein. In 1948, the estimate was advanced to 255,000 after the 1940 formula was applied to the later population figures. These estimates would seem to indicate a trend of increasing blindness in this country. But whether it is real or statistical is anybody's guess.

It is undoubtedly true that the number of elderly blind is increasing, for between 1940 and 1950 the number of persons over sixty-five advanced almost 20 percent. Within that same decade, there was an increase in blindness among children born prematurely, but Dr. Hurlin does not feel that that has reached a point which would invalidate his estimate. The higher ratio of 1953, 198, seems more realistic than the 175 of the 1940 estimate in comparison with England's ratio of 175 with a less generous definition of blindness.

Most of the continental European countries have fairly complete reports of the extent of blindness owing to their highly developed programs of social welfare, but, because only persons with extreme visual loss are included, the reported incidences of blindness are low. A glance at the Oxford report reveals Germany reporting 53 per 100,000; Switzerland, 58; Finland, 72; Norway, 75; Sweden, 91; and Denmark, 98. It is hard to explain the two highest reports received—Eire, 233, and Northern Ireland, 300—except by attributing them to the magnanimous emotions of the Irish.[7]

Other available statistics direct attention to countries with very high ratios, especially in areas where endemic causes of blindness, such as trachoma, onchocerciasis, and loss of sight from smallpox are still prevalent. For these countries, any adequate statement of either incidence or total number is almost beyond estimation. In China, it is estimated that there are over 2,000,000 blind persons, making a ratio of 450 per 100,000; while the estimated two million in India gives a ratio of 500. Egypt, once called the country of the blind, reported 85,622 in 1937, with a ratio of 530.

The highest incidence of blindness of which there is record is in the Jinja area (upper reaches of the Nile) where it is 4,187 per 100,000. This is due to ocular onchocerciasis, caused by infection with the filarious worm *Onchocerco volvulus*, which is transmitted by the fly *Simulium damnosum*, or "buffalo gnat"; there is no known cure for the disease except the eradication of the fly. High rates, ranging from 500 to 1500 per hundred thousand, are to be found in other parts of Africa.

Any attempt to state the number of persons throughout the world who come within some definition of blindness must necessarily be an estimate. The League of Nations, in its study of 1929, stated

that, out of a total population of 763,867,565 in the countries dealt with, there were 801,443 blind persons, or 104 per 100,000 of population . . . The United States Census in *The Blind in the United States, 1910*, page 11, attempted a very rough estimate of the total blind population of the world and obtained 2,390,000, but added, "probably this is an understatement . . . Other estimates have been made up to 6,000,000 and it is possible that, if the standard of blindness was everywhere an economic one, the total would be not much, if any, less than the latter estimate." [8]

The World Health Organization of the United Nations has prepared a report on The Prevalence of Blindness, issued in January 1953. This is undoubtedly one of the most comprehensive studies ever made; it deals with many countries, uses all available statistics, and states when possible the definitions applied. Some of the data unfortunately are not as up to date as one would wish; nevertheless, the figures have sound validity for an area where estimation is the only recourse.

To estimate the total number of blind in the world is a hazardous task, since the sources of information vary greatly . . . and the national figures are all more or less rough approximations . . . An estimate is nevertheless shown . . . Asia with about 52 percent of the world's population has more than 70 percent of the total number of the blind . . . Africa has the highest prevalence rate. The lowest prevalence rates are found in Europe and Oceania . . . By applying these computed rates to the total population of each continent around 1950, an estimate of the total blind population has been obtained. On this basis, the number of blind persons in the world is around 6.6 millions.[9]

On the basis of the statistics that were returned on the questionnaires of the study made in 1950 by the Department of Social Affairs of the United Nations,[10] the incidence of blindness in the nations covered would seem to be about 330 per 100,000, or a total number of 5,898,000 blind persons. Applying this ratio to the total population of the world, there is an indication that the number of blind persons might be 6,700,000.

These figures, however, are stated with great reluctance, because of the limited information available and incompetence to deal with the facts adequately. Their validity is further questioned because in many countries the criteria on which they are based is not known. In the reports of countries with a tremendous amount of blindness, concern is probably only for the truly blind, those who cannot see; while in the countries with good social-welfare programs there is a broader concern for those with limited vision.

There are these general conclusions to be drawn: that there will be low incidences of visual impairment among children and high incidences among the aged in countries with high standards of living, efficient medical care, and good schemes for the sightless; whereas in countries having no social-welfare programs and limited facilities for the blind, plus low standards of living, the reverse situation will be true. These facts go to show that blindness is no longer to be considered primarily from an emotional angle nor studied merely as a physical problem, but that it has important social aspects which demand earnest attention and present a challenge to the social conscience of the world.

17 CAUSES AND CURES
OF BLINDNESS

To know that at the present time, at a very minimum, more than six million people in the world are considered to be blind is a challenge far exceeding that which confronted the encyclopedists of France nearly three centuries ago. They and their followers took up the challenge of their time and through education and economic aid did much to alleviate the sordid condition of the sightless. Today the physical scientists exceed in potentiality the philosophers and to them the blind rightly turn for release from their imprisoning darkness.

To make any adequate presentation of these possibilities is difficult, in fact, almost impossible, because of the unknown etiology of so many and the lack of definite diagnosis of their physical disability. And yet in the area of causes and cures great gains have been achieved, for blindness is a sense deprivation that is readily apparent and, as has been pointed out, easily defined in terms of visual loss and economic handicap.

In this consideration of causes and cures of blindness, the approach will be more historical and social than medical or surgical. It is desired to indicate that, in addition to the restricted lives of those visually handicapped, society in general pays a heavy price for its tolerance of the loss of sight and its reluctance to take strong measures toward its prevention. More than fifty years ago a distinguished authority said that one-third of all blindness should have been prevented, one-third might have been prevented, and only one-third was inevitable. Since that time, there have been notable advances in the unceasing efforts aimed toward the ultimate conquest of blindness.

Looking at the whole matter historically, the cause of blindness that stands out above all others through the ages is trachoma. And although it still prevails in some areas, trachoma has been effectively banished in many parts of the world. "True trachoma" has been defined as "a world-wide serious and important ocular infection, generally of long duration, characterized by the presence of trachoma bodies or granulations." It is now considered to be a virus infection and loss of vision is due to the scarring of the cornea, to exposure and ulceration of the cornea, and to the results of secondary infection.

Trachoma is to be found in all parts of the world where people live crowded together under unhygienic conditions, and it is easily transmitted through public baths, towels, clothing, or other forms of contact. In countries where heat is great and flies are numerous, they can be factors in spreading the disease. If the infection is treated early enough, the prognosis is favorable, and today, through modern drugs, loss of sight can be prevented if the eye has not been too severely damaged.

Tradition places the origin of trachoma in the Valley of the Nile, and for a time it was known as "Egyptian ophthalmia." There is definite evidence of its existence in that country nearly 3500 years ago. The papyrus exhumed by the German Egyptologist, Georg Ebers, in 1872, dating about 1550 B.C., has references to the disease and prescriptions for its treatment. With due incantations, a solution with copper, myrrh, and cyprus seeds as the main ingredients was to be applied to the patient's eyes with a goose quill.

It is surmised that trachoma existed in both India and China in ancient days, and there is reference to it in early Greek records. When, during the famous retreat under Xenophon in 400 B.C., 10,000 Greeks became blind, it was conjectured that it was caused by Egyptian ophthalmia, but this is not sustained, for it is now considered that the more likely cause was snow blindness. Military expeditions, however, proved to be the medium that spread trachoma from the country of its origin, until it become the scourge of Europe during the early part of the nineteenth century.

Napoleon's expedition to Egypt landed on July 1, 1798. After the capture of Cairo, the victorious French troops were stopped, not by the enemy, but by disease. As July was the seasonal height for trachoma, there is every evidence that this was the potent force which proved greater than British arms. However, when the French troops left Egypt in 1801, they did not spread the eye disease that made them helpless, for trachoma was not as widely known in France at that time as it was in other countries. This was probably due to the fact that Napoleon's troops were not immediately disbanded.

The English troops that went to Egypt in 1800 were almost all attacked by trachoma, and when they returned home in 1803 the contagious eye disease was carried with them. Immediately disbanded, the troops returned to their homes and trachoma spread until it became a national emergency. A military asylum intended for 1400 orphans of soldiers was crowded with 1500 cases of trachoma in 1811, and in 1818 there were 5000 cases in England, and the government voted £100,000 for the support of the victims.

About the same time, this form of ophthalmia was found among the troops of Belgium. A German ophthalmologist called in for consultation recommended that the infected men be discharged and sent home. Soon trachoma spread through all of that country. Austria, on the other hand, acted more wisely. There, not only were victims of trachoma retained in the army, but recruits were accepted with this eye ailment. Isolated in a single hospital for a four-month course of treatment, 80 percent were cured and the country was spared the scourge of other lands.

The Prussian army, however, suffered most. "Never in the memory of man was any army," wrote a regimental surgeon in 1839, "even the French of Egypt, so terribly ravaged by disease, as the Prussian army during the years 1813 to 1820." [1]

Between those years, 25,000 men in the Prussian army had trachoma, 1100 becoming totally or partially blind. Italians, in contact with the French soldiers from Egypt at Elba and Leghorn, were soon infected. In Italy, the climax came in 1813. The disease did not strike the Russian army, however, until later. During the period from 1818 to 1839, 76,000 cases were reported.

From this terrific experience, trachoma became known as "military ophthalmia," but the fundamental causation was not military, but the crowded conditions of army barracks life, the common towels and drinking cups, and other unsanitary factors that in modern life have been discarded. And wherever such contaminating factors as close common living, inadequate sanitary arrangements, and lack of medical care continue, the incidence of trachoma will be high, especially in the crowded marts of warm countries.

While there are some indications that there were a few cases of trachoma in the United States in colonial days, it was not until early in the nineteenth century that the disease was at all widespread. As shiploads of people were coming to the new land at the time trachoma was ravaging Europe, it would be expected that some of them would bring over the ocular infection. When immigration reached its peak in the second half of the century, trachoma become a serious menace. Toward the end of the century (1897), a law was enacted prohibiting entrance into this country of any persons showing evidence of trachoma. The United States Public Health Service screened all arrivals on ships from Europe and set up programs for control of the disease. These were so effective that the incidence was reduced from 4 percent prior to 1897 to 2 percent in 1915, and trachoma is now in the United States a negligible causative factor of blindness.

For some unexplained reason, trachoma was first found among the mountaineers of Tennessee, Kentucky, and West Virginia and along the Mississippi River, as early as 1825. Its presence there was attributed to "itinerant laborers and the indolence of people." Another strange aspect is that Negroes are immune to trachoma while the American Indians are its most tragic victims. The United States Public Health Service reported that it had encountered only one band of Indians, a group of forty-six scattered along the north shore of Lake Superior, wholly free from trachoma, while another examination of 39,000 Indians showed that 17 percent were affected. Among these, the incidence ranged from 70 percent in Oklahoma to 0.2 percent in New York State.

When it was revealed that the disease was least prevalent among Indians living in the open of the reservations and most prevalent among inmates of Indian boarding schools, owing undoubtedly to the poor living conditions, the United States Public Health Service inaugurated in the early 1920's a program to control trachoma among the Indians by going to the source. A railroad car equipped with clinic facilities, beginning in the Ozark region of Missouri, rolled over the tracks giving treatments and operations wherever groups could be assembled. In 1923, the mobile clinic reached Rolla and there it settled down and developed into the notable Trachoma Hospital now conducted by the State of Missouri.

Hospitals were also set up in most of the Indian reservations and, although trachoma still persists in some areas, it is no longer a menace even among the Indians. The drive against trachoma has become more effective through the use of the sulfonamide drugs. Although some physicians still place more confidence in the older methods, Dr. Arthur A. Sinescol, head of the Missouri Trachoma Hospital, claims "In my opinion, at least, trachoma responds to treatment with the sulfonamide drugs more quickly and with less injury to the affected tissue than to the use of any other drug previously used." [2]

Conquest of this potent cause of impaired vision requires the concerted action of medical and social forces wherever conditions conducive to infection with it are found. The problem now, both here and abroad, is to put to use the modern methods that will prevent loss of vision in those affected and eliminate the breeding places of this disease. Already some progress is being made. Even in Egypt, the country of its origin, trachoma has been greatly reduced.

From 1917 to 1947, the incidence was cut from 1.3 to 0.052 percent through the efforts of mobile teams of physicians, nurses, and sanitary engineers. In 1950, the Ministry of Health put into operation 106 new units, and ophthalmologists were sent to Mecca and Medina to examine and treat the eyes of the pilgrims.

Israel, through the activities of the Hadassah Anti-Trachoma Services, had brought about the virtual eradication of trachoma by the end of 1947, but the later mass migrations of refugees into that country resulted in a reappearance of the disease. Over 63,000 cases were reported in 1953. Of the immigrants from Yemen, 79.83 percent had trachoma. Among those from North Africa, the incidence was 13.19 percent while among those from Europe, there was the low ratio of 1.20 percent. The great proportion of the cases were among children living in the rural immigrant settlements. With government help, Hadassah is attempting to cope with the problem.

In Iran, where in some towns in the southern part of the country the incidence of trachoma is as high as 90 percent, a tremendous drive is being made to eliminate this cause of visual defect. The city of Teheran, in the northern part, has cut the incidence of trachoma among school children from 40 percent in 1931 to 2 percent in 1949, through school clinics, with necessary operations and treatments in the Eye Hospital, and with social workers clearing up conditions in the homes. In the southern area, a demonstration project sponsored jointly by the Imperial Organization of Social Welfare and the Near East Foundation was carried out in 1949–1950 in the town of Dizful by six Austrian physicians, assisted by nurses and sanitary engineers. Starting with one-fifth of the town, individuals were given medical and surgical care, the ancient public baths and privies were destroyed, modern conveniences were provided, and the whole area was sprayed with DDT. So successful was the effort that plans were made to extend the work.

Most of the work so far in the Middle East has been to cure the persons involved and to change the environment in which trachoma thrives. The first large-scale attempt to attack this dread disease fom the standpoint of prevention is to be undertaken by the Harvard University School of Public Health under a grant of $500,000 from the Arabian American Oil Company. The program is to find a vaccine that will provide immunity and thereby cut down the millions of its victims in eastern countries. The Harvard research group will work in Boston and the Middle East. The study will also go into all phases of infectious eye disease, including factors affecting recovery and immunity.

With trachoma well under control or practically eliminated in the West, the World Health Organization is now concentrating on its banishment in the Near East, where endemic trachoma still persists. Spot checks and sample surveys reveal the danger areas, and plans for definite projects are being completed. In 1950, WHO felt optimistic enough to state:

Trachoma is no longer universal. When a people has a high standard of hygiene and the medical body is sufficiently numerous . . . if the national campaigns already under way are continued and coördinated, they will meet with vigorous international support. Our generation may perhaps witness the disappearance of trachoma.[3]

Optimistic about the conquest of trachoma, WHO is now turning attention to other forms of endemic ophthalmia. At a United Nations meeting in New York on January 7, 1953, the World Health Organization representative reported:

The virus infection trachoma, though very wide-spread throughout the region, is believed to be far less important as a cause of blindness, [because] uncompleted trachoma may result in spontaneous cures in 60 percent of the cases; it also responds to modern chemotherapy and antibiotic therapy, though more slowly than the purulent ophthalmias.[4]

The so-called purulent ophthalmias are now causing WHO more concern than trachoma, for the report states that they cause 80 percent of the cases of blindness in the areas under study, and are overwhelmingly the more important because they "cause destructive lesions with great rapidity giving rise to permanent defects and immediate treatment is essential. Fortunately, they respond to modern methods of treatment, especially chemotherapy and antibiotic therapy." "Again," the report states, "the weapons are available; their application is a question of administration."

Chief among the purulent ophthalmias is ophthalmia neonatorum, a Latin term meaning "inflammation of the eyes of the newborn," which in this country is more commonly called "babies' sore eyes." This may be defined as "an inflammatory disease of the conjunctiva, usually appearing within the first few days of life and generally due to the action of microorganisms." There are several forms of this disease. One, known as Koch-Weeks, due to simple catarrhal vaginitis, is not of frequent occurrence, whereas cases due to gonococcus are the most common. Of other possible forms, staphylococcus follows gonococcus in frequency. This infection of infants' eyes in its several forms has been recognized from the dawn of medicine. The ancients administered to the inflamed eyes of infants drops of oils of various kinds with little success, and even today this cause of blindness has increased until in some countries the World Health Organization considers it a greater menace than trachoma.

Fortunately, however, a happier story can be told in other parts of the world, for "babies' sore eyes" in all countries with good medical programs and high health standards is almost entirely eliminated. In England in 1879, 25 percent of all blind children lost their sight from ophthalmia neonatorum, whereas now "no child need ever again be blind from this cause, but a few will still continue to do so until it is possible in England to ensure attention from a nurse, midwife, or doctor at every birth." [5] At the beginning of this century, this infection was the largest single cause of blindness among children in the United States. In 1907, 28.2 percent of loss of sight was attributed to this cause; in 1932, it was reduced to 7.0 percent; and in 1950, it was down to 1.2 percent.

The story of how this conquest has been achieved is in itself an interesting one, illustrating as it does the potential power of careful and continuous research. In this case, however, the good result was attained largely through trial and error and without the meticulous attention and scientific facilities that are now available in the field of research. As early as 1750, a German physician pointed out that the cause of this blinding disease was not within the eyes of the newly born child, but came through their contamination from the mucus found in the birth canal of the mother.

This led to many attempts to find a solution that would offset the damaging effect of the diseased mucus. In 1807, Benjamin Gibson, an English physician, proposed washing the eyes of the newborn child with a liquid calculated to remove the offending matter or to prevent its noxious action. Another English physician named Hagus in 1879 advised that the eyes be wiped free from every trace of moisture the instant the head was born and before the baby had time to open his eyes.

On January 16, 1822, the Saxon minister of health gave instructions to midwives that the eyes of newly born children be washed with a fine linen rag dipped in clean water, and then, realizing the contagiousness of the infection, suggested that after doing so, each midwife should wash her hands with water in which carbolic acid or some disinfectant was mixed. Another approach to the problem was made in 1837 when it was proposed by the Spanish Cortes "to enjoin that infants should be baptized in warm water, as it was believed that ophthalmia resulted from the chill incurred in the performance of that rite." [6]

In 1873, a German physician attempted to cure the affected eyes by dropping a solution of 1 percent of silver nitrate into the eyes of children at birth. This reduced the incidence in the year 1875–1876 from 5.6 to 2.6 percent. Ten years later, another German physician claimed to have reduced the incidence 3 percent by washing the eyes with pure water. Reports of the use of silver nitrate for "babies' sore eyes" soon reached the United States, but they were not well received, at least in Boston.

Dr. Hasket Derby, father of the late distinguished ophthalmologist Dr. George Derby, when he returned to Boston in

1875 from medical studies in Germany, became an ardent advocate. "Fresh from von Graefe, Arlt, and Donders, he felt that he represented," so he wrote later, "the rising sun of science and even apt to believe that all knowledge was concentrated in his own person." [7] With that self-assurance the youthful Derby rebuked the senior professor of ophthalmology at the Harvard Medical School, Dr. Henry W. Williams, for his admonition to physicians to avoid the use of silver nitrate.

This, Dr. Williams had written, was of no more value than a common practice of some nurses who felt that they accomplished wonders "by squirting into the eyes a stream of breast milk; a waste of valuable material, but a procedure which does no other harm." Silver nitrate, he felt, was too caustic for infants' eyes, and so he asked "the profession to let the babies off easy." [8] To which Dr. Derby retorted, "We are adjured to 'let the babies off easy.' If we go a step further and apply this precept to their moral training, we are met by a remonstrance from the wisest king of Israel. The sting of the caustic though sharp is temporary, its results most salutary, as each may ascertain for himself." [9]

While speculation and discussion concerning the use of silver nitrate as a preventive agent were occupying obstetricians and ophthalmologists both here and abroad, a German physician was quietly carrying on a careful study which was rewarded by finding the right solution. This was Dr. Karl Siegmund Franz Credé. Born in Berlin, December 23, 1819, he received his professional degree in 1842 and from 1843 to 1850 was associated with the Banks Obstetrical Clinic in Berlin. In 1856, he went to Leipzig to be professor of obstetrics at the university in that city and director of the Leipzig Lying-In Institution and School for Midwives. Here he remained until his death on March 14, 1892.

While working in Leipzig, Credé made the study that led to the discovery of the proper solution of silver nitrate to be used successfully in preventing ophthalmia neonatorum. For thirteen years, from 1870 to 1882, he examined 4,057 babies at the time of birth, 318 of whom, or 7.8 percent, developed ophthalmia neonatorum. On the basis of this observation, and probably through experimental work with several medicines, Credé finally arrived at the decision that a single drop of 2-percent solution of silver nitrate simply dropped into the baby's eyes as soon as convenient after birth would destroy the noxious effects of the mucus and would do no harm to unaffected eyes.

For three years following this decision, the German physician examined 1,160 children and had only one case of ophthalmia neonatorum. On the basis of this study, Dr. Credé in 1881 made the first announcement of his findings. This was later followed by his final treatise on the subject, published in 1884. The importance of these reports rests largely on the fact that, based on such extensive study and coming from so eminent an obstetrician, they excited considerable medical attention. So thorough was Dr. Credé in his study that his procedure, recommended in 1881, is still considered standard and in many countries its administration is required by law. The social significance of this great discovery was the simplicity of its application and the certainty of the cure.

While more recently some of the new miracle drugs are being tried, most obstetricians are hesitant to give up a cure that has proved to be so effective over so many years and through which the sight of millions of children has been saved. "Though only an obstetrician," states the writer of Credé's brief biography in the *American Encyclopedia and Dictionary of Ophthalmology,*

he will always walk with the great company of distinguished physicians, and hundreds, nay possibly even thousands, of other ophthalmologists whose own ungestated eyes are yet to be washed by the magical solution. For Credé did more, much more, than merely to bring back sight to the blind. To a large degree he succeeded in vanquishing the unspeakable monster of blindness from the very face of the earth! [10]

There are other widespread causes of visual impairment, many of which, although greatly reduced, are yet far from conquered. Smallpox, once a large causative factor, is now practically eliminated in countries using the vaccine developed by Dr. William Jenner in England in 1798. This was the forerunner of other preventive vaccines, culminating most recently in the Salk vaccine for polio, which have been potent factors in the conquest of crippling diseases. Because of the reduction of tuberculosis, loss of sight from that dread disease is no longer of grave concern.

Syphilis, still a potent factor in all parts of the world, is gradually being reduced by modern cures and preventive measures. WHO reports that in the Near East it is intense only in certain areas. In the United States in 1941, 15 percent of all blindness was attributed to this disease. Among children in schools for the blind, there has been a notable decrease. In the twenty years from 1930 to 1950, the rate of blindness from syphilis dropped 80 percent. "Now that the attention of the public generally is focused on the problems of syphilis," writes Dr. Conrad Berens, "we may hope that the control of this disease will eventually eradicate blindness and visual impairment from this cause." [11]

Acquired syphilis can be accurately diagnosed in its early stages and cured. The former prolonged treatment has now been considerably shortened through the use of the miracle drugs. Congenital syphilis may likewise be brought under control through systematic treatment. It is now generally accepted that the disease may be averted in the children of infected mothers if properly administered treatments are begun as early as possible, and in any case not later than the fourth month of pregnancy. The routine requirement of premarital blood tests and prenatal tests are forward and hopeful steps. The time may be approaching when the request, made by a father to his prospective son-in-law when he asked for his daughter's hand, will also be routine: "Come over next week and let us talk about it, and when you come, bring along a record of your Hinton test."

Another field, where perhaps the responsibility for permitting continued loss of sight falls more heavily upon those now blind than upon those who have sight, is blindness attributed to hereditary causes. Without question, much might be accomplished if it were possible to exercise control in this field. It would be very easy, but equally ineffective, to point out that all loss of sight from hereditary causes could be eliminated in one generation if those whose blindness is of that nature would refrain from the bearing of children in whom the defects would be carried on. And yet it must be definitely understood that this is an area where the burden falls on the present generation of blind people and where they may, if they have a sense of social responsibility, make a positive contribution to the social goal of the conquest of blindness.

A considerable reduction of blindness from hereditary causes does lie within the realm of possibility and should be effected. Much information about hereditary blindness is now available. Dr. J. Myles Bickerton of England stated, "We know more about the hereditary diseases of the eye than about those of any other organ, and for the good reason that, being the most important and complicated of our sense organs, its slightest defects cause marked disturbances of functions." [12]

The importance of attack in this field lies in the fact that Dr. Bickerton estimated that 24 percent, or nearly one-quarter, of all blindness is from hereditary causes. Dr. Harry Best of the United States lists causes totaling slightly less than 30 percent, but adds that "it is difficult to know with exactness just how much of this blindness is of a hereditary character." [13] More recent studies, however, would place the extent of hereditary blindness at lower ratios and it is probable that in both of the above references some of the causes included are congenital rather than hereditary. Dr. Best is on surer ground when he adds: "This problem presents a serious situation and deserves full attention." [14]

Another cause of blindness that is perhaps more social than medical is the damage to sight as a result of accidents. Considerable progress has been made in this field, although accidents are still rated in this country as the cause of about 15 percent of all blindness. From 1936 to 1950, however, there was a 30 percent drop in blindness resulting from accidents among children. A number of factors contributed to this encouraging decline—legislation to control fireworks and air guns, enforcement of these laws by local and state police, general safety education both through publicity and through discussions at parents' meetings led by public health nurses, social workers, and blindness prevention officers. Nevertheless, in 1953, approximately 100,000 eye injuries occurred among our youngsters, 1200 so severe that the sight of one or both eyes was lost.

In the adult area there has also been considerable progress. Although an estimated 300,000 eye accidents occur annually, there has been a decrease of 40 percent in the past ten years. A large part of this is due to the Safety First campaigns that for the last twenty years have been promoted among most of the large industries. These campaigns encourage the conscientious wearing of safety glasses at times when there is possibility of eye injury. In an effort to promote wider use and appreciation of these safety devices, the National Society for the Prevention of Blindness has been sponsoring what is known as the Wise Owl Club. This Club admits to membership only those industrial workers whose sight has been saved by the wearing of safety glasses. Since its founding in 1947, 7000 men and women have become members of the exclusive Wise Owl Club, and more than a thousand of them have had the sight of both eyes saved. In preserving their own sight, they have saved industry nearly $30,000,000 that would have been paid in compensation, in addition to the saving of loss of income and the cost of rehabilitation of the individuals themselves.

These devastating causes of blindness may be considered primarily as social problems, for they require coöperative social action for their control and conquest. While there is a certain historical interest in them among many people, too often there is no real concern about them. Yet all of these causes strike individuals and these forms of blindness may come into any home. Even in this country there is still some trachoma in a zone running through the central states from the Alleghenies to Kansas and Oklahoma, and the disease has been so prevalent among the American Indians that special hospitals are still maintained in some of the reservations to cope with it.

Ophthalmia neonatorum still manifests itself because of neglect or carelessness in administering drops at the time of birth in too many children, and the "social diseases" have an insidious way of appearing where least expected, owing too often to lack of compulsion in seeing that the available cures and preventives are put to work. Accidents will continue to happen, and war, even cold war, darkens forever the lives of too many young men. No conquest over evil in any form is easily achieved, but in the arena of ophthalmology advances are being made and they will continue so long as medical and social forces muster their resources for the fray.

18 THE CONQUEST
OF BLINDNESS

THE conquest of blindness in this country, and in fact in all parts of the world, is often deterred by the apathy of too many people toward its social implications and a detached confidence that "it cannot happen in my home." Despite the progress that has been made through modern methods of restoring vision and expanding plans for the prevention of blindness, possible loss of sight still hovers over many people. During the period of this writing, the National Society for the Prevention of Blindness had a car card among the many that form a frieze in trolleys and trains. Displayed in bold type was this question: "Will blindness strike your home?" The card then continued, "At least 750,000 Americans now living will be overtaken by blindness" and it advised: "1. Know the facts; 2. Protect your sight; and 3. Support eye research."

These stark statements, in addition to warning those who read them that loss of sight may happen in their homes, outline an approach to further consideration of the causes and cures of blindness. This will be done here from the individual rather than the social point of view, and, to make the picture a little more graphic, these causes will be presented according to the age of the persons affected and will include only the major forms of loss of sight.

One of the most striking aspects of this presentation is the seeming trend toward more blindness as a result of the dramatic advances of modern medicine in saving and prolonging human life. There are more blind children today because of success in keeping alive more premature babies. There is an increasing number of old people, many of whom become blind, for one of the significant social phenomena of this generation is the fact that people live longer and therefore anything associated with old age assumes greater proportions.

The cause most prevalent among older people is cataract, a cloudiness of the lens inside of the eye caused by the degeneration of the lens fibers. Usually attributed to the normal deterioration associated with old age, this condition of the eye may also result from injury or from a chronic infection in the person involved. While this form of visual impairment seems to be increasing, the advance is probably due largely to increased life expectancy. The social significance of this eye defect is that it is remediable. In the incipient stage of cataract, improvement in visual acuity may occur under appropriate general treatment.

Ophthalmologists are able through operations to remove the clouded lens in severe cases and to prescribe spectacles that take over the focusing power. Experiments are now being made with plastic lenses that can be placed within the eye. Older people beginning to experience a blurring of vision would do well to consult an ophthalmologist promptly. Dr. Conrad Berens tells of a study made in England in which cataract was shown to be the most prevalent cause of blindness and that "if it had been possible to make the examinations at an earlier date, operation probably would have restored the vision of many patients." [1]

Coming to middle age, the form of blindness which strikes most frequently during these years is that due to glaucoma. Occurring usually after the age of forty, glaucoma causes about 12 percent of all adult loss of sight. Its causes are unknown and it strikes insidiously, often without the victim having any idea that he is going blind because the onset is gradual and central vision is not greatly affected in the early stages.

Often called "the mystery disease of ophthalmology," it is now being treated as "a sick eye in a sick body," for investigators are beginning to believe that general disorders and chronic infections may play an important role. In its earliest stages, glaucoma can be controlled, but it cannot be cured, and if left too long may lead to complete blindness.

The teen-age group reveals a cause of blindness only recently observed. This is found among that growing company of young people who have diabetes and who, though kept alive through the use of insulin, seem to be vulnerable to kidney disorders and loss of sight. This, however, is not due to the treatment but rather to its lack or inadequacy. Boston's eminent physician, Dr. Elliott P. Joslin, a pioneer in the use of insulin, claims: "We can prove that loss of eyesight or kidney maladies can be deferred or prevented if diabetic treatment is followed faithfully."

Among the 1,500,000 diabetics in this country, there are some for whom the diagnosis came too late for full control; others, especially teen-agers, slip up on their treatments, and many of them arrive at schools for the blind. An interesting side light on this situation and one that supports the frequent suggestions of regular eye check-ups is that an ophthalmologist can often, by his observation of the retina through the ophthalmoscope, detect diabetes long before the patient is aware that he has the disease.

In the years of childhood, excluding infancy, barring accidents and delayed manifestations of either congenital or inherited causes, there are today certainly fewer reasons and less need for blindness. It is true that chemical intoxication, meningitis, and tumors can and do cause loss of sight, but the incidence is slight. Of extreme importance in this age group is the early detection of cross eyes and of squint. Even if only one eye is affected, there is always the danger that, if the good eye is damaged later, there will be another blind child.

Accidents, although reduced 30 percent from 1936 to 1950, still take too heavy a toll among children. Three out of four of the eye injuries in this age group occur during unsupervised play. Junior-high-school pupils are especially prone to eye accidents, and boys injure their eyes three times as often as girls. Among children, blindness from fireworks is being reduced through control of sales, but too many children's eyes are being popped out by BB guns, and legislation to prohibit their sale seems hard to secure and more difficult to enforce.

Blindness among children from scarlet fever and measles is now practically unknown. Seventy-five years ago, they were listed as chief causes among the pupils at Perkins Institution. There are, however, two diseases already described that have congenital forms. These are glaucoma and cataracts. Congenital glaucoma occurs in infancy; it is characterized by the bulging of the eyeball and is often called buphthalmos or "ox eye." Little can be done for the condition, and often the eye is removed because of pain or secondary complications. Congenital cataract, if extensive, may interfere seriously with vision, but if partial, there may be little disturbance. There is considerable evidence that many cases are hereditary, and it has recently been learned that toxic substances administered to the mother during pregnancy may lead to cataract in the offspring.

The first reports of this form of blindness among children came from Australia in 1941. Later it was confirmed in this country that when a prospective mother contracts rubella, or German measles, there is a high possibility that her offspring will have cataracts at birth. The risk of deformity is now estimated at about 17 percent if infection occurs during the first three months of pregnancy, and 12 percent during the second three months. This is encouraging because the original statistics indicated that more than 80 percent of the offspring of mothers who had rubella during pregnancy came into the world with a defect of the heart, ears, or eyes. Even the decreased incidence makes many feel that it would be advisable for girls to have German measles early in life rather than to expose their prospective children to the possible consequences of this disease.

Coming to the years of infancy, an entirely new cause of blindness, and one of the most contradictory and enigmatic that has ever been found in the history of ophthalmology, is now causing grave concern. This is a disease usually confined to babies who are prematurely born and who weigh less than

4 pounds at birth. Within this group a number of the infants will have their sight impaired, some to the point of total blindness, within six months of birth. This cause of visual impairment was first discovered by the late Dr. Theodore L. Terry in February 1941, as he was about to operate on a six-months-old boy for what had been diagnosed as cataract. As a result of his early studies the Boston ophthalmologist named the new disease retrolental fibroplasia, which means a fibrous mesh behind the lens.

More recent studies, however, reveal that this is primarily a disease of the retina and of the vitreous humor which starts as an unexplained distortion and overgrowth of the blood vessels of the retina and is followed by separation of the retina and the formation of an opaque mass behind the lens composed of detached retina, blood vessels, and fibrous tissue. In general, the disease cannot be observed until from three to five weeks after birth and at the end of the fourth or fifth month the process ceases and the child is liable to visual impairment, according to the degree of retinal detachment and the extent of the fibrous mesh that has formed.

Recognition of the disease is too recent and the diagnostic criteria are not yet defined with sufficient clearness to make reports from various clinics fully comparable. These reports, however, do indicate wide variations both in the rates of incidence and in the degrees of severity. More recent studies reveal that there is a mild form as well as a severe form. At first, the investigators were chiefly concerned with cases in which the sight was lost or severely affected. Later studies, however, indicate that the milder-seeming forms of the disease also cause eye damage. Children who during infancy had only a slight indication of retrolental fibroplasia were found upon reaching school age to have seriously defective vision. On the other hand, some of the children who showed the most severe form in infancy are, at school age, finding a considerable amount of useful vision. This is due to another strange aspect of this disease, an unexplained regression of the condition which leads to more sight.

A confusing aspect of this strange disease is the fluctuation ber of cases were reported in Geneva, Switzerland, in 1949, but in the summer of 1953, Zurich claimed to have no cases. Up to 1945, England claimed to have no cases, but in October 1953, 51 percent of the children in the Sunshine Homes for preschool children were reported to have been blinded by retrolental fibroplasia. In the summer of 1953, Paris reported that between 8 and 9 percent of premature children had severe cases of retrolental fibroplasia; and Sweden, which reported its first case in 1948, has found through a recent study that thirty-eight infants born between 1945 and 1950 had lost their vision owing to retrolental fibroplasia.

Concern for this new form of blindness began with the first case discovered by Dr. Terry. Money was soon made available through the Foundation for Vision for extensive research which has been carried on continuously at the Massachusetts Eye and Ear Infirmary, working in conjunction with the Boston Lying-In Hospital and more recently with the Children's Medical Center in Boston. Notable work was soon under way at the Wilmer Clinic at Johns Hopkins Hospital, followed by research in New York, Washington, and Chicago. The Kresge Institute in Detroit later organized extensive research facilities.

Now nearly all obstetricians and ophthalmologists are on watch for manifestations of this strange malady. In 1952, all of the groups interested in the problem joined in a coördinated study that includes centers of research in eighteen hospitals. By sharing research findings and distributing the areas of investigation, definite progress has been made toward determining the causative factor, although there is every indication that nothing can be done to recover the sight of the 8000 children who are already its victims.

After exploring many possible causes, all of which led to negative results, the many investigators came to the positive conclusion that oxygen is the chief causative factor. Concentration on this resulted in three schools of thought concerning the part played by oxygen as it was administered to newborn infants in incubators. One group claimed that the disease developed as a result of oxygen deficiency. Another school felt that it was the high concentration of oxygen which caused the eye damage, and that the rise in incidence of retrolental fibroplasia corresponded to the increase in the use of oxygen in hospitals to assure the survival of premature babies.

The third and most recent group concluded that "prolonged high oxygen administration is an important factor in the development of retrolental fibroplasia." This conclusion was based on the accumulating evidence that the incidence of the disease was generally lower in hospitals where either no oxygen was used or it was administered infrequently. One of the earliest observations of the relation between the amount of oxygen administered and the frequency of eye damage was made in 1949 by the group at the Massachusetts Eye and Ear Infirmary, after a study of the records of premature infants born at the Boston Lying-In Hospital from 1938 to 1948. They found that the infants in whom retrolental fibroplasia subsequently developed had received longer oxygen therapy than those in whom retrolental fibroplasia did not develop. This observation was confirmed later by groups in Australia and England, who reported a higher incidence of retrolental fibroplasia in hospitals that used oxygen liberally than in hospitals that used it sparingly.

The extensive administration of oxygen to premature babies while in incubators is the result of improved equipment for its use. When it was learned that it kept alive many infants who might not have survived without it, oxygen was given in generous measure. It has now been established that there is no significant difference in mortality rates between infants in the low- and the high-oxygen groups. Because of this it is now felt that it can be safely recommended that the use of oxygen therapy be rigidly restricted to infants who show a definite clinical need for it and that it no longer be used as a routine treatment for premature babies. This has led to a program of more careful regulation of this form of therapy and its overuse is being cautiously avoided.

In the public announcements implicating oxygen as the cause of retrolental fibroplasia, there is an inherent danger that many will feel that the full solution of the problem is to be found in discouraging the "routine" use of that agent and all that remains is to train hospital personnel in the controlled administration of oxygen. This is definitely important, steps in that direction are being taken, and it is expected that there will be a drastic reduction in the frequency of this condition, but it must not be forgotten that there may always be occasional babies who require oxygen for survival, and for these safe methods of administration must be worked out. However, some investigators, especially in the United States, feel that while oxygen is the major causative factor, there may be other causes as yet unrecognized.

The attempts in England, in Sweden, and in this country to reproduce the disease in animals through continuous high oxygen treatment have resulted in eye damage that closely resembles *mild* retrolental fibroplasia. Because of this, the group in Boston, where research in this field originated, raises these questions: "Does excessive oxygen therapy actually cause the mild disease as it does in animals, or does it produce severe disease by aggravating already existing mild cases which are the result of some other cause? Is it possible that any one of a number of ailments to which premature infants are susceptible, which perhaps themselves create a need for oxygen therapy, might give rise to the mild disease?"

And other investigators suggest that perhaps the occurrence of retrolental fibroplasia is less directly related to oxygen therapy than to the state of health or the low gestational age which gives rise to the need for oxygen therapy. Determination of these, as yet unrecognized, factors is one of the present concerns of research in this field and the answers must be found before this strange disease can be written off as an interlude in the advance of ophthalmic history.

"This disease," wrote Ida Mann and Antoinette Pirie, "which is an unnatural disease, a disease of civilization—for uncivilized premature babies would find no incubators handy and would die—is being tackled and solved in a highly reasonable and scientific way." [2] The English writers are perhaps overhopeful in thinking that this unnatural disease is being scientifically solved in any way and their description of it as a disease of civilization is an oversimplification of the problem. But it may be that they have touched on an aspect that is more natural and fundamental than those stressed in the early scientific research.

For some time, most of the investigators of the disease maintained that the rate of survival of prematurely born infants had not materially advanced. A study of the records of the Boston Lying-In Hospital, however, revealed that there has been from 1937 to 1952 a threefold increase in survival. If this advance is confirmed by the records of other hospitals with high rates of retrolental fibroplasia and the incidences are correlated with survival rates, it may be affirmed that this unnatural disease, as the English writers call it, may be more natural and normal than has been thought.

This, of course, does not in any way relieve the medical profession of the need for continued research. In fact, it makes it more imperative because the end sought is not an explanation of the cause of loss of sight but its assured prevention. Present developments will undoubtedly alter the direction of future studies and may lead to the conclusion that a more hopeful solution is to find ways of preventing the premature birth of all infants. For it may well be that this form of impaired vision, with its wide variations from total blindness to slight damage, its unique intensification and regression, and its strange geographical spotting, is one of the by-products of the great medical advance of modern civilization in somewhat the same way as the survival and blinding of some victims of diabetes.

All of this leads to the last admonition on the display card of the National Society for the Prevention of Blindness: "Support eye research." There is great need, not only for the money to carry on the work, but for the training of competent persons to conduct modern research. For quite a long time, persons interested in the blind have been advocating that consideration be given to the conquest of blindness rather than to increased and more expensive programs for alleviating the lot of the blind. While blind persons should have every provision needed to compensate for their handicap, society in general should see the wisdom of supporting a program of prevention rather than being content with a system of alleviation.

There is some encouragement in this area also, for during the past few years more and more money has been made available for research in blinding diseases. A few years ago, the advocates of this type of program claimed that less than $400,000 a year was spent upon research in blindness. This rose to $905,000 in 1949 and to $1,579,000 in 1952, a 75-percent increase, or approximately $5.00 per blind person. But this sum, large as it may seem, is less than 1 percent of what was spent during the same year for education, rehabilitation, and relief for the blind.

Without question, the most significant and hopeful development in the agelong attempt to understand and to control blinding diseases has been the opening of the Clinical Center at the National Institutes of Health in Bethesda, Maryland. Conducted by the United States Public Health Service and supported by federal funds, the new Institute of Neurological Diseases and Blindness has already initiated a strong program of research. A plan of making grants for research to nonprofit institutions and of fellowships to individuals for training in the methodologies of research was soon under way. The Institute also provides grants to support graduate training in medical schools and hospitals and clinical traineeships to individuals for specialized training in neurological diseases, ophthalmological diseases, and rehabilitation.

Established by the Congress in August 1950 under Public Law 692, the Institute was granted in 1952 its first appropriation of $1,250,000 which enabled it to function on a "stand-by" basis. "But in 1953 the seriousness of neurologic disorders and blindness as a public health problem began to be acknowledged; the Institute's appropriation was increased by 225 percent. Again in 1954 the 1953 appropriation was almost doubled and its program was definitely 'off the ground'; its research productivity was surging at a remarkable rate." [3] In 1955 the Institute was supporting eighty projects in eye research in twenty-one states. Its grants in eye research advanced from $10,000 in 1951 to $80,000 in 1955. Training grants in ophthalmology have been made to eight medical schools and two hospitals. In August 1955 a clinical unit was opened at the Institute for investigation of ophthalmic disorders.

In the field of specific blinding diseases the Institute undertook to support research in three areas; glaucoma, uveitis, and retrolental fibroplasia. Concerning the last project, Dr. Pearce Bailey, Director of the Institute wrote:

> The preliminary findings of the retrolental fibroplasia study have now emerged and there can be little doubt that the results constitute the most important single clinical advancement in ophthalmology during the past decade. The findings were unequivocal that oxygen—the oxygen routinely administered to premature infants in their incubators—was definitely associated with the cause of retrolental fibroplasia and that oxygen, therefore, should be administered to premature infants only in times of severe clinical crises . . .
> The 8000 children already blinded by retrolental fibroplasia will, during the course of their normal life span, cost the states, the federal government and several welfare organizations $100,000 each for their education, training and support, or a total of $800,000,000. But after their lifetime, the tragedy of long life without sight because of retrolental fibroplasia will have virtually ceased and so will the heavy economic burden to the nation.[4]

Three points in this program should be emphasized. First, the inclusion of blindness with the study of neurological diseases. The importance of this is that, as has been pointed out earlier, one of the largest causes of loss of sight is the atrophy of the optic nerve—a person may have a perfectly good eye and yet not be able to see because of the defective optic nerve. This is purely a neurological problem, but essential in overcoming blindness. The second is that, along with direct research, there is a plan to train workers in the medical and technical fields. And the third, and perhaps the most forward-looking, is the provision for clinical traineeship grants to persons interested in rehabilitation.

Social concern for the problems of blindness and its alleviation cannot cease with full understanding of the medical aspects and the possibility of cures and preventives but should seek to culminate in the rehabilitation of the individuals involved and to aim at their restoration to society as contributing members. While workers for the blind need to understand more fully the medical aspects of their rehabilitation clients, medical men must come to know and to accept the economic possibilities of blind persons. But with the progress that has already been made, it may not be too much to hope that medical research combined with physical rehabilitation and social acceptance will bring fulfillment of the words of the Old Testament prophet Isaiah: "I will bring the blind by a way they knew not. I will lead them in paths which they have not known. I will make darkness light before them and crooked places straight. These things will I do and not forsake them."

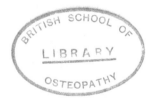

References

1. SHOOTING STARS ON THE HORIZON

1. Homer, *The Iliad and Odyssey*, trans. William Cowper (Boston, 1814), III, 185–186.
2. *The Poems of Ossian*, trans. James MacPherson (New York, 1810), II, 78–79.
3. Will Durant, *The Age of Faith* (New York: Simon and Schuster, 1950), p. 266.
4. R. A. Nicholson, *Translations of Eastern Poetry and Prose* (Cambridge, England, 1922), p. 102.
5. John Milton, *Works* (New York: Columbia University Press, 1931), II, part I, p. 79.
6. Ishbel Ross, *Journey Into Light* (New York: Appleton-Century-Crofts, 1951), p. 62.
7. Maurice Maeterlinck, *The Life of the Bee* (New York, 1907), pp. 12–14.
8. Michael Anagnos, *Education of the Blind* (Boston, 1882), p. 4.
9. Denis Diderot, *Early Philosophical Works*, trans. Margaret Jourdain (Chicago and London, 1916), p. 77.
10. M. de la Sauvagere, "Accomplishments of a Blind Lady," *London Magazine* (May 1762), p. 267; also *Massachusetts Magazine* (January 1789).
11. Diderot, *Early Philosophical Works*, pp. 152–154.

2. BEGINNINGS WITH CHILDREN

1. Michael Anagnos, *Education of the Blind* (Boston, 1882), p. 14.
2. *Ibid.*
3. Maurice de la Sizeranne, *The Blind as Seen Through Blind Eyes*, trans. F. Park Lewis, M.D. (New York, 1893), p. 58.
4. Richard S. French, *From Homer to Helen Keller* (New York: American Foundation for the Blind, 1932), p. 81.
5. Margaret Goldsmith, *Franz Anton Mesmer* (New York, 1934), chap. 6, on Marie Theresa Paradis.
6. French, *From Homer to Helen Keller*, pp. 73–74.
7. Ishbel Ross, *Journey into Light* (New York: Appleton-Century-Crofts, 1951), p. 118.

8. Samuel Gridley Howe, "Education of the Blind," *North American Review*, 37:16 (1883).

3. STIRRINGS IN EUROPE

1. Samuel Gridley Howe, *Address of the Trustees to the Public* (Boston: New England Institution for the Education of the Blind, 1833), pp. 6, 7, 10.
2. Samuel Gridley Howe, *Forty-Third Annual Report of Perkins Institution* (Boston, 1874), pp. 137–138.
3. Gabriel Farrell, ed., *The Education of Blind Youth*, Report of the Proceedings of the International Conference of Education of Blind Youth, Bussum, Holland, July 25 to August 2, 1952.
4. Gabriel Farrell, "Social Aspects of Blind Children"; A survey made for the Department of Social Affairs, United Nations, 1950. (Not published; copy available at United Nations and Perkins Institution Library.)
5. Farrell, *The Education of Blind Youth*, pp. 117–118.
6. *Report of International Conference of Workers for the Blind*, Merton College, Oxford, England, August 4–12, 1949 (New York: American Foundation for the Blind; London: National Institute for the Blind, 1951), pp. 133–134.

4. PIONEERING IN AMERICA

1. Laura E. Richards, *Samuel Gridley Howe* (New York and London: Appleton-Century, 1935).
2. George Ticknor, *Life of William Hickling Prescott* (Boston, 1864), p. 235.
3. James G. Mumford, *Surgical Memoirs* (New York, 1908), p. 251.
4. Laura E. Richards, ed., *Letters and Journals of Samuel Gridley Howe* (Boston, 1909), II, 13–14.
5. Samuel Gridley Howe, *Forty-Third Annual Report of Perkins Institution* (Boston, 1874), p. 38.
6. Mumford, *Surgical Memoirs*, p. 255.
7. *Ibid.*, p. 248.
8. Merle E. Frampton and Ellen Kerney, *The Residential School* (New York: New York Institute for the Blind, 1953), p. 2.
9. *Report of the New York Institute for the Blind* (New York, 1845), p. 5.

5. OPENING OF NEW WAYS

1. Laura E. Richards, ed., *Letters and Journals of Samuel Gridley Howe* (Boston, 1909), II, 104–105.
2. George F. Meyer in Helga Lende, ed., *What of the Blind?* (New York: American Foundation for the Blind, 1938), I, 85.
3. Samuel Gridley Howe, *Eighteenth Annual Report of Perkins Institution* (Boston, 1850), pp. 42–43.

4. Samuel Gridley Howe, *Nineteenth Annual Report of Perkins Institution* (Boston, 1851), pp. 14–16.

5. Samuel Gridley Howe, *Address at the Laying of the Corner Stone of the New York State Institution for the Blind* (Boston, 1866), pp. 38–39.

6. Edward Jarvis, *Thirty-Sixth Annual Report of Perkins Institution* (Boston, 1867), pp. 8, 10.

7. Edward Jarvis, "Letter to Samuel Gridley Howe," *Thirty-Seventh Annual Report of Perkins Institution* (Boston, 1868), p. 23.

8. Michael Anagnos, "Workshops for the Blind," *Proceedings of the Ninth Biennial Meeting of the American Association of Instructors of the Blind* (New York, 1886), p. 25.

6. THE WAY AHEAD

1. Edward E. Allen in Helga Lende, ed., *What of the Blind?* (New York: American Foundation for the Blind, 1938), I, pp. 52, 55.

2. George F. Meyer in P. A. Zahl, ed., *Blindness* (Princeton: Princeton University Press, 1950), pp. 110, 111.

3. Thomas D. Cutsforth, *The Blind in School and Society* (New York: American Foundation for the Blind, 1951), pp. 201–202.

4. William M. Cruikshank, as quoted by V. R. Carter, "Where Shall Blind Children Be Educated?" *International Journal for the Education of the Blind*, 4:22 (1954).

5. *Report of the Committee on Education of Partially Seeing Children* (New York: National Society for the Prevention of Blindness, 1952; Publication 149), pp. 3–6.

6. Walter R. Dry, "Coordination of the Residential School with the Public School," *Outlook for the Blind* (September 1948), pp. 207–208.

7. Edward J. Waterhouse, "The New England Plan," *The Lantern* (June 1952), pp. 6–8.

8. Samuel Gridley Howe, *Forty-Third Annual Report of Perkins Institution* (Boston, 1874), pp. 119–120.

7. CHILDREN OF THE SILENT NIGHT

1. J[ohn] B[ulwer], *The Deafe and Dumbe Man's Friend* (London, 1648), p. 142.

2. *Hablar el Idioma Español* (Madrid, 1759), I, 264.

3. Quoted by Charles E. H. Orpen, *Anecdotes and Annals of the Deaf and Dumb* (London, 1836), p. 338.

4. Samuel Gridley Howe, *Ninth Report Respecting the New England Asylum for the Blind* (Boston, 1840), p. 25.

5. Anna G. Fish, *Perkins Institution and its Deaf-Blind Pupils, 1837–1933* (Watertown, Massachusetts, 1934), p. 32.

6. Helen Keller in Helga Lende, ed., *What of the Blind?* (New York: American Foundation for the Blind, 1938), I, 156–157.

7. Malcolm J. Farrell, "A State Facility for the Blind Retarded," *Outlook for the Blind,* 49:168 (May 1955).

8. FINGERS FOR EYES

1. Pierre Villey, *The World of the Blind* (New York, 1930), p. 18.
2. *Ibid.,* p. 39.
3. Jean Roblin, *The Reading Fingers, Life of Louis Braille,* trans. Ruth G. Mandolian (New York: American Foundation for the Blind, 1955).
4. W. H. Illingworth, *History of the Education of the Blind* (London, 1910), pp. 17–18.
5. J. M. Ritchie, *Concerning the Blind* (London, 1930), pp. 51–52.
6. Quoted in *ibid.,* p. 66.
7. *Ibid.*

9. BATTLE OF THE TYPES

1. *First Report of the Pennsylvania Institution for the Instruction of the Blind* (Philadelphia, 1833), p. 5.
2. *Second Report of the Pennsylvania Institution for the Instruction of the Blind* (Philadelphia, 1835), p. 8.
3. Samuel Gridley Howe, *Fourteenth Annual Report of Perkins Institution* (Boston, 1846), p. 19.
4. *Ibid.,* p. 45.
5. Perkins Institution, correspondence file, 1868.
6. W. H. Illingworth, *History of the Education of the Blind* (London, 1910), p. 46.
7. *To the Trustees, Principals and Teachers of Blind Asylums,* Proceedings of in Appendix to the *Fifth Biennial Report,* Missouri Institution for the Education of the Blind (St. Louis, 1886), p. 7.
8. Sir Clutha MacKenzie, *World Braille Usage* (Paris: UNESCO, distributed by Columbia University Press, 1953).

11. EARS FOR FINGERS

1. *The Optophone* (Jersey City, N.J.: The Federated Engineers Development Corporation, October 1921), p. 11. Pamphlet; copy in Perkins Institution Library.
2. George W. Corner in P. A. Zahl, ed., *Blindness* (Princeton: Princeton University Press, 1950), pp. 439–440.
3. Clifford M. Witcher, "Some Communication Aspects of Visual Prosthesis" (unpublished paper, Research Laboratory of Electronics, Massachusetts Institute of Technology, 1953).
4. Thomas A. Benham, "Evaluation and Development of a Guidance Device for the Blind," paper read before the American Association for the Advancement of Science, December 1953.
5. George W. Corner, in *Blindness,* p. 433.
6. *Ibid.,* p. ix.

12. COMPENSATION—THE EARLY OBJECTIVE

1. J. M. Ritchie, *Concerning the Blind* (London, 1930) , p. 130.
2. *Ibid.*, p. 134.
3. *Ibid.*, p. 135.
4. *Report of International Conference of Workers for the Blind* (New York: American Foundation for the Blind; London: National Institute for the Blind, 1951) .

13. PARITY—THE PRESENT GOAL

1. Samuel Gridley Howe, *First Annual Report of New-England Asylum for the Blind* (Boston, 1833) , p. 5.
2. Richard S. French, *From Homer to Helen Keller* (New York: American Foundation for the Blind, 1932) , pp. 249–250.
3. Edward Everett Hale, *Proceedings of the Public Meeting on Behalf of the Printing Fund for the Blind* (Boston, 1881) , p. 17.

14. THE TOLL OF WAR

1. Sir Arthur Pearson, *Victory over Blindness* (New York, 1919) , p. 14.
2. *Ibid.*, p. 20.
3. Harry Best, *The Blind* (New York, 1919) , p. 694.
4. *Ibid.*, p. 695.
5. Col. J. H. King, Jr., "Army Ophthalmology," *Military Surgeon*, 112:88 (February 1953) .
6. Lloyd Greenwood in P. A. Zahl, ed., *Blindness* (Princeton: Princeton University Press, 1950) , p. 262.
See also Zahl, ed., *Blindness*, chaps. 17–20.

15. WHO ARE THE BLIND?

1. John Milton, *Sampson Agonistes* (New York, 1931) , I, part II, p. 340.
2. I. Mann and A. Pirie, *The Science of Seeing* (Harmondsworth, England: Penguin Books, 1950) , p. 20.
3. *Ibid.*, pp. 91–92.
4. Herman Snellen, *The Methods of Determining Acuity of Vision in Diseases of the Eye*, ed. Norris and Oliver (Philadelphia, 1897) , p. 15.
5. Arnold Sorsby, *History of Ophthalmology* (London: Staples Press, 1948) , p. 74.
6. Snellen, *Methods*, p. 11.
7. "Estimations of Loss of Visual Acuity, Report of Committee of Sections of Ophthalmology, American Medical Association," *Archives of Ophthalmology*, 54:463 (September 1954) .
8. Snellen, *Methods*, p. 13.
9. T. S. Sze, World Health Organization, personal letter to author, 6 August 1953.

16. THE EXTENT OF BLINDNESS

1. Arnold Sorsby, *The Causes of Blindness in England and Wales* (London: H. M. Stationery Office, 1950; Memorandum No. 24), p. 30.
2. *Welfare of the Blind* (Geneva: Series of League of Nations Publications, III, Health, 1929), p. 20.
3. Department of Commerce, Bureau of the Census, *The Blind in the United States, 1920* (Washington, 1922), pp. 9–10.
4. Sorsby, *Causes of Blindness*, p. 21.
5. *Ibid.*, p. 22.
6. R. G. Hurlin, *Estimated Prevalence of Blindness in the United States* (New York: American Foundation for the Blind, 1953), p. 7.
7. *Report of International Conference of Workers for the Blind* (New York: American Foundation for the Blind; London: National Institute for the Blind, 1951).
8. *Welfare of the Blind,* pp. 24–25.
9. "The Prevalence of Blindness and Deaf-Mutism in Various Countries," *The Epidemiological and Vital Statistics Report* (Geneva: World Health Organization, 1953), VI, part I, pp. 14–15.
10. Gabriel Farrell, "Social Aspects of Blind Children," A Survey made for the Department of Social Affairs, United Nations, 1950. (Not published; copy available at United Nations or Perkins Institution Library.)

17. CAUSES AND CURES OF BLINDNESS

1. J. Boldt, *Trachoma,* trans. J. Herbert Parsons and G. Treacher Collins (London, 1914), p. 14.
2. Arthur A. Sinescol, "Trachoma," *Archives of Ophthalmology,* 42:431 (1949).
3. "Trachoma," Report of the World Health Organization, *Sight Saving Review,* 20:124 (Summer 1950).
4. "Blindness in the Middle East," Paper read at United Nations Meeting, New York, 7 January 1953 (Geneva: World Health Organization, 1953), p. 5.
5. I. Mann and A. Pirie, *The Science of Seeing* (Harmondsworth, England: Penguin Books, 1950), p. 20.
6. Sidney Stephenson, *Ophthalmia Neonatorum* (London, 1907), p. 160.
7. Hasket Derby, "Personal Recollection of Graefe, Arlt and Donders," *Archives of Ophthalmology,* 2:255 (1929).
8. "Henry W. Williams Correspondence," *Boston Medical and Surgical Journal,* (1875), p. 291.
9. Hasket Derby, "Personal Recollection," p. 389.
10. Thomas H. Shastid, "Karl Siegmund Franz Credé," *American Encyclopedia and Dictionary of Ophthalmology* (Chicago, 1914), V, 3557.
11. Conrad Berens in Helga Lende, ed., *What of the Blind?* (New York, 1938), I, p. 27.

12. J. M. Bickerton, "The Inheritance of Blindness," *Eugenics Review*, 24:115 (July 1926).

13. Harry Best, *Blindness and the Blind in the United States* (New York, 1934), p. 67.

14. *Ibid.*, p. 78.

18. THE CONQUEST OF BLINDNESS

1. Conrad Berens in Helga Lende, ed., *What of the Blind?* (New York, 1938), I, p. 23.

2. I. Mann and A. Pirie, *The Science of Seeing* (Harmondsworth, England: Penguin Books, 1950), p. 128.

3. Pearce Bailey, "America's First National Program in Eye Research," *American Journal of Ophthalmology*, 40:123 (July 1955).

4. Pearce Bailey, "Clinical Success with Three Eye Conditions," *Outlook for the Blind* (June 1955), p. 222.

INDEX

Abdu'l Ala al Ma'arri, 8
Accidents, causing blindness, 232–233, 237–238
Accommodation of eye, 197, 201
Achievement tests, 40
Adult blind, 146, 163
Africa, 218, 225
Akerly, Dr. Samuel, 49
Alabama School for the Deaf and Blind, 87
Al-Ashar, University of, Egypt, 147
Alcorn, Sophia, 86
Allen, Edward E., 119; at Pennsylvania Institution (1890–1906), 52; at Perkins (1906–1931), 63–65
Alphabets, 6, 24; embossed, 24; manual, 83, 85; string, 95
Alston, John, 101, 108, 118
Amblard, Henri, 195
American Association of Instructors of the Blind, 59, 113, 161
American Association of Workers for the Blind, 112, 113, 161
American Asylum for the Deaf, Hartford, 80
American Bible Society, 109
American Blind People's Higher Education and General Improvement Association, 161
American Braille, 104, 111–112, 119
American Braille Press, 176
American Committee on Uniform Type, 113–114
American Foundation for the Blind, 130, 131, 144, 162, 190; and education, 58, 69; and deaf-blind, 89–90; and type, 113–114, 124–125; statistics, 215

American Foundation for Overseas Blind, 162–163
American Lodge, Torquay, England, 183–184
American Medical Association, 203, 206
American Printing House for the Blind, Louisville, Kentucky, 70, 127
American Red Cross, 181
Anagnos, Michael, 13, 18, 127; at Perkins (1876–1906), 62–63
Analyzing Reader, 137
Anne, Queen of England, 11, 120, 123
Anocaloscope, 132
Anrep-Nordin, Madam Elizabeth, 88
Armanni, Vincent, 13
Armitage, Thomas Rhodes, 34–36, 153; and braille, 103–104, 112
Army, U.S., 174, 185, 211
Asia, 4, 146; blindness in, 217–218
Ascertainment of blindness, 211–219; notification, 211–212; census, 211–213; registration, 214–215; estimation, 215–217
Association for the Chinese Blind, 163
Association of Teachers of the Blind, England, 161
Astigmatism, 197
Asylum, 60, 146–148, 150, 152. See also Schools
Asylum and Industrial School for the Blind, Bristol, England, 31, 102
Asylum for the Industrious Blind, Edinburgh, 153
Atkinson, J. Robert, 103
Australia, disease in, 240

Austria, 104, 120, 200, 209, 222; education in, 27–28, 32, 45, 89
Avon Old Farms Convalescent Hospital, Connecticut, 186–187
Awl, Dr. William, 53

Babies, blind, care of, 71–72, 182
Babies' sore eyes. *See* Ophthalmia neonatorum
Bacon, Roger, 200
Bailey, Dr. Pearce, 246
Baker, Col. E. A., 129
Banks braille writer, 122
Banks Obstetrical Clinic, Germany, 229
Barbier, Charles, 96–99, 114, 118
Barden-LaFollette Bill, 168, 184–185
Bards, blind, 5
Barr and Stroud, Ltd., Glasgow, 133
Barrett, James, 80
Batavia, New York, state school, 70
Beach, Albert Ely, 121–122
Beggars, blind, 4, 17, 146, 148, 149, 199
Belgium, 32, 176, 222; Bruges, 151; New Ordinance of Ypres, 151
Belisarius, 173
Bell, Alexander Graham, 82, 122
Bell Telephone Laboratories, 136
Benham, Prof. Thomas A., 140–141
Berans, Dr. Conrad, 231, 236
Berkeley, Bishop, 14
Best, Dr. Harry, 179, 232
Bible, 3–4, 247; editions for blind, 102, 106, 108–109
Bickerton, Dr. J. Myles, 232
Bifocals, 200
Blacklock, Thomas, 30–31
Bledsoe, John F., 65
Blinded Veterans Association, 194
Blind Persons Act of 1920, England, 156
Blindness, prevalence of. *See* Statistics
Blind retarded, 90–92
Bohemia, school in Prague, 32
Books for the blind, development of uniform type for, 96–117; printing, 101, 106, 108–109, 124–128; distribution, 108, 129; libraries, 127–128, 130; mailing, 129; aids to

reading, 143; public funds for, 70, 126–128, 155, 164
Boston Line Type, 106–109, 110
Boston Lying-in Hospital, 240, 241, 242
Brace, Julia, 80
Bradley, Omar N., 192
Braille, 98–100, 103–104, 105, 110–117; variations of, in English, 110–115; World Conference of Work for the Blind, 114–115; spread throughout world, 115–117; World Braille Conference, 117. *See also* Line type; Moon type; Type for blind
Braille, Louis, 97–100, 105, 121
Braille Institute of America, 103, 126, 127
Braille Writer (Hall's), 119–120
Brain, 198
Braun, Jacob, 27
Bridge North, Oldbury Grange, England, 184
Bridgman, Laura, 49, 78, 80–82, 83, 84, 85, 88
Brieux, Eugène, 175
Brisac, J., 175
British and Foreign Blind Society, 34
Brush Development Company, Cleveland, 140
Bryan, Frank C., 126
Bulwer, Dr. John, 78, 86
Buphthalmos, or ox eye, 238
Bureau of Public Assistance, 205
Burt, William Austin, Typographer, 121
Bussum Conference, Holland, 37–40, 129

Café Saint Ovide, 19, 23, 41, 148
California, 185; School for the Blind, 59, 86, 87; nursery in, 71
Campbell, Francis J., 34–36
Campbell, Guy, 35
Canada, 211; Montreal, 187
Cane, use of, 142, 187
Cardan, Jerome, 94
Carter, Abby and Sophia, 46
Cataracts, 12, 14–15, 168, 236, 238
Causes of blindness, 220–234 *passim;*